Dr. Bhiti's Book

How Incurable Diseases Can Be Treated with Food Elimination

by

Somsak Bhitiyakul, M.D., FACP

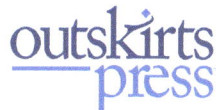

How Incurable Diseases Can Be Treated With Food Elimination
All Rights Reserved.
Copyright © 2021 Somsak Bhitiyakul, M.D.
v3.0

The opinions expressed in this manuscript are solely the opinions of the author and do not represent the opinions or thoughts of the publisher. The author has represented and warranted full ownership and/or legal right to publish all the materials in this book.

This book may not be reproduced, transmitted, or stored in whole or in part by any means, including graphic, electronic, or mechanical without the express written consent of the publisher except in the case of brief quotations embodied in critical articles and reviews.

Outskirts Press, Inc.
http://www.outskirtspress.com

ISBN: 978-1-9772-1789-9

Cover Photo © 2021 Somsak Bhitiyakul, M.D. All rights reserved - used with permission.

Outskirts Press and the "OP" logo are trademarks belonging to Outskirts Press, Inc.

PRINTED IN THE UNITED STATES OF AMERICA

The reader of this book will understand illnesses, how they come about, and how to treat them. This will be explained in a simple language for everyone to understand. This is an easy guide to prevent conditions such as strokes, heart attacks, lung disease, and kidney disease, as well as controlling abdominal ailments, premature kidney failure, and diabetes mellitus. The book will also discuss autoimmune diseases, such as systemic lupus erythematosus, rheumatoid arthritis, Sjögren's syndrome, and how to take care of your hips, knees, and other joints. In addition, the book will also describe a diet to cure ulcerative colitis, Crohn's disease, psoriasis, and psoriatic arthritis.

The purpose of this book is to expand the knowledge of dietary management and see how it affects different illnesses. Dr. Bhitiyakul will describe his treatment plan by avoiding food that is harmful and suggesting a minimal use of prescribed medications. All readers planning to change their diet based on suggestions in this book should first consult their primary care physician.

The book represents the real communication between Dr. Bhitiyakul and his patients; these are his ideas. He does not represent any persons other than himself or any organizations.

Table of Contents

About the Author i

Chapter 1: The Aging Process and Atherosclerosis 1

Chapter 2: Kidney Diseases and How to Protect the Kidneys 3

Chapter 3: IgA Nephropathy and Focal Segmental
Glomerulosclerosis . . . Curable Diseases? 5

Chapter 4: My Autoimmune Diet: No Cow Products. No Shellfish ... 20

Chapter 5: Diabetes Mellitus and Kidney Failure 22

Chapter 6: Urination 24

Chapter 7: Autoimmune Diseases: SLE and Rheumatoid Arthritis .. 26

Chapter 8: Sjögren's Syndrome and Reversible Kidney Failure 67

Chapter 9: Polymyalgia Rheumatica (PMR). Why Am I So Weak? 69

Chapter 10: Fibromyalgia 71

Chapter 11: What Causes Breast Cancer, Lung Cancer,
Colon Cancer? Certain Molds 72

Chapter 12: Heart Problems 74

Chapter 13: Thickened, Calcified Sclerotic Heart Valve,
Pulmonary Hypertension, and an Enlarged Heart . . . to
Reorganize the Phase of Heart Disease before It Gets Worse 77

Chapter 14: Another Case of Diffuse Thickening (Sclerosis)
on the Aortic Valve Cusps 83

Chapter 15: Hypertension—Pay Attention 89

Chapter 16: Lung Problems 91

Chapter 17: Chest and Lungs 92

Chapter 18: Abdomen 95

Chapter 19: Stool 104

Chapter 20: Yeast and Mold Allergies 106

Chapter 21: Psoriasis and Psoriatic Arthritis 113

Chapter 22: Improvement of Degenerative Disease of the
Large Joints and Spine . . . Is It Real? 115

Chapter 23: Herpetic Neuralgia 117

American College of Physicians-American Society of Internal Medicine

Presents To

Somsak Bhitiyakul

the

Ralph O. Claypoole, Sr. Memorial Award

for Devotion of a Career in

Internal Medicine to the Care of Patients

Given in the City of Philadelphia, this eleventh day of April, two thousand and two.

William J. Hall
President

CHAPTER 1

The Aging Process and Atherosclerosis

When we are young, anything we eat will generally make our bones and muscles grow. After a meal, food is absorbed, and phosphorus rises in our bodies and stimulates the production of the parathyroid hormone. This hormone from the parathyroid gland will help administer calcium and phosphorus toward bone growth and, shortly thereafter, will shut down when it's done.

When people reach the age of 60, the parathyroid hormone tends to be produced continuously and production does not stop as it should. This creates a situation where calcium and phosphorus are deposited throughout the body in soft tissue, such as arterial walls, tendons, skin, heart valves, etc. Atherosclerosis increases, and bone strength decreases. The bones get thinner as the arteries get thicker and narrower. Therefore, as we get older, we should avoid phosphorus-rich foods, such as dairy, eggs, meat, poultry, whole grain items, and carbonated soft drinks.

Vitamin D is significant to stabilize the parathyroid hormone and regulate its production. If Vitamin D deficiency occurs, the parathyroid hormone level will be hard to control. It is essential to keep the Vitamin D level regular.

Atherosclerosis can be accelerated by many diseases, such as hypertension, diabetes mellitus, hypercholesterolemia, smoking, and obesity. Strenuous exercise is also not always beneficial because it will cause the blood pressure to go up, developing an enlarged heart while arteries harden. This will accelerate the aging process, so it needs to be controlled. Therefore, moderate exercise is recommended.

Atherosclerosis will cause organs to malfunction, leading to strokes, heart attacks, kidney failures, and artery insufficiency of the legs and arms. It will also cause people to age quicker as they become reliant on using a cane, walker, and wheelchairs.

Our body tissue sustains damage all the time. Our organs have a lot of wear and tear that requires ongoing repairs to maintain organ function. Just like in our homes, we need to repair and take care of maintenance issues. If we need to fix a roof, we buy the proper materials and repair it to prevent further damage to our homes. Similarly, our bodies need repair work as well. Our DNA determines our repair work by issuing the proper amino acid sequence to make tissue repairs. However, the person needs to take the proper food supplements and amino acids in order to repair damaged tissue and prevent further damage.

CHAPTER 2

Kidney Diseases and How to Protect the Kidneys

The disease that promotes fear for both patients and nephrologists is massive leg edema and very high blood pressure affecting people of all ages. This disease does not respond to currently recommended treatments, and it slowly damages the kidneys, eventually requiring dialysis in a few years. However, this can be regulated through diet restriction with good results. Please see the case presentation beginning in 2001.

The kidney's primary function is to maintain homeostasis by the selective retention or elimination of water, electrolytes, and other solutes.

How do we know if we have kidney problems? The beginning of a kidney problem is generally asymptomatic. There might be an issue with urination (increased frequency, painful, lengthy time to urinate, evidence of blood in the urine), back pain at night, swelling of both legs, puffy eyes, and a swollen face.

A blood test for BUN, creatinine, and routine urinalysis is generally good enough to screen for kidney disease. The urinalysis should have no proteins, no blood, no sugar, and no leukocyte esterase.

To protect the kidneys:

1) See a kidney specialist (nephrologist) for diagnosis and treatment.
2) Treat hypertension effectively, preferring a BP of 120/70 at the physician's office, not measured at home.
3) Diabetes mellitus, either type 1 or type 2, should have A1c<7.0, and the patient should be taking an angiotensin-converting enzyme inhibitor (ACEI) or angiotensin receptor blocker (ARB).
4) Do not smoke.
5) Reduce cholesterol to LDL<100.
6) Treat kidney stones that develop from ulcerative colitis and Crohn's disease with diet restrictions.
7) Check your homocysteine and bring it down to normal.
8) If there is a prostate enlargement that causes partial or total blockage of the bladder outlet, seek treatment to prevent hydronephrosis (swollen kidneys), leading to kidney damage.
9) Treat urinary tract infections effectively to prevent kidney infections.

CHAPTER 3

IgA Nephropathy and Focal Segmental Glomerulosclerosis . . . Curable Diseases?

IgA nephropathy and focal segmental glomerulosclerosis affect people of all ages. Both diseases cause the kidneys to leak proteins and/or blood into the urine. A normal functioning kidney will not leak either into the urine. Proteinuria is a condition where protein is present in the urine. The presence of either protein or blood may indicate kidney damage or disease. This may potentially lead to hypertension, leg edema, and, eventually, kidney failure. People younger than 30 years old generally end up on dialysis if they have either disease. Treatment typically consists of several medications and/or an immunosuppressive agent. In my experience, neither is effective, and the patient eventually needs dialysis within 3 to 4 years.

Over the years, I have found that dietary change can be significant. I will recount the history of two patients.

Michael O. was diagnosed with IgA nephropathy at 55 years old with 5 gm proteinuria and severe hypertension. He was put on a strict diet and told to avoid all cow products and shellfish. Within 2 months, there was a significant improvement in his bloodwork; he had lower proteinuria and improved serum creatinine. Serum creatinine was

1.4, which was slightly elevated (normal 0.76–1.27). A high level of creatinine will indicate kidney disease. Now, 17 years later, his creatinine is 1.67, and his 24-hour urine protein is 717.6.

Mrs. B was diagnosed with IgA nephropathy at the age of 69 after her kidney transplant. She was also put on a strict diet avoiding cow products and shellfish. She continued to take her usual Prograf and prednisone. Within 2 months, there was also improvement in her bloodwork. Her kidneys are functioning well with creatinine at 1.35 as of December 2016. Her creatinine at the time of her biopsy was 2.9.

Diet restriction seems to stabilize either disease over a long time. My recommendation is that the patient be treated with whatever medication the physician chooses but to add the dietary restrictions as well. Once the disease is under control and manageable, discontinue the medication and keep the diet in place. The physician should request 24-hour urine collection for protein every 2–3 months and check the patient's urine for blood or heme presence. If there is positive blood or protein in the urine, the physician should question the patient about his/her diet, specifically inquiring about cow and shellfish products. Once cow and shellfish have been completely eliminated, it will take 3–4 weeks for the urinary protein to come down.

The Disappearance of Proteinuria and Stabilization of Kidney Function through Diet

by

Somsak Bhitiyakul, M.D. FACP
Ralph O. Claypoole Sr. Memorial Award Recipient 2002
Graduate of Chulalongkorn University, Bangkok, Thailand
Founder of Kingston Hospital Dialysis Center, Kingston, NY

and

Saharat Bhitiyakul, M.D.
Internal Medicine, Board Certified, & Hypertension
Graduate of Albany Medical College

368 Broadway, Suite 201
Kingston, NY 12401
(845) 339-5811
Abstract

Background:

The disappearance of proteinuria and stabilized kidney function for more than 10 years following diet manipulation. The author is a nephrologist who is taking care of patients following kidney transplantation. Some of his patients who had ESRD due to either IgA nephropathy or focal segmental glomerulosclerosis and post-transplantation kidney function became deteriorated but appear to have stabilized kidney functions following the elimination of cow products.

Methods:

Case #1:

Virgin case of FSGS kidney biopsy with an electron microscope revealed focal segmental glomerulosclerosis (Dr. Gerald B. Appel, Professor of Nephrology, Columbia University College of Physicians and Surgeons thought that we were unable to exclude IgA nephropathy) with 5 g protein in the urine and blood pressure 170/110. The patient was told to eliminate cow products and shellfish since February 2001. No immunosuppressive agent was given.

Result Case #1:

Proteinuria slowly decreased and down to normal. The patient maintained his kidney function until now. This is a 12-year follow-up.

Case #2:

Second Case of IgA nephropathy in a kidney transplant. Two years 4 months after transplantation, the creatinine went up to 2.95 with conventional kidney transplantation therapy. Kidney biopsy on the transplanted kidney revealed IgA nephropathy. Diet intervention was added to the regimen.

Result Case #2:

Her creatinine slowly came down to 1.19 on 10/15/12. As far as I know, this is the first known case in any transplantation program.

Conclusion:

Two cases of biopsy-proven IgA nephropathy with significant proteinuria and microscopic hematuria maintained their kidney function and the disappearance of proteinuria over a 10-year follow-up. Successful story.

The author is very grateful for the advice of Gerald B. Appel, M.D., Professor of Nephrology, Columbia University College of Physicians and Surgeons, for diagnostic certainty of these cases. He kindly read the patient charts with me on November 19, 2012.

Case #1:

Michael O., born in 1946, a rural New York State auto mechanic and volunteer fireman. A 6-foot, 254-pound white male, BMI 34. On a routine fireman yearly physical examination, his PCP found heavy proteinuria 5.218 gram in a 24-hour urine collection (2001), microscopic heme-positive urinalysis, hypertension 170/110 mmHg. PCP started him on Accupril 20 mg and quickly referred him to see me. He was previously in good health. He was found to have a small amount of blood in his urine 3 years earlier and was told that he probably passed a kidney stone, but no medication was given, and he was asymptomatic.

I saw him on 2/9/2001. He is a nonsmoker, nice gentleman, white, muscular male. I quickly add atenolol 50 mg, Norvasc 5 mg, and increased Accupril 40 mg daily. A few weeks later, his blood pressure came down to 126/80, and a kidney biopsy was done on 4/3/2001. The kidney biopsy found focal mesangial sclerosis with scattered electron dense deposits suggestive of focal segmental glomerulosclerosis.

However, there is no tissue for a direct immunofluorescence study. The pathologist diagnosed that most consistent with focal segmental glomerulosclerosis (kidney biopsy with light microscopic exam and electron microscopy done at Albany Medical Center, Albany, N.Y.). Dr. Appel thought that this biopsy is unable to exclude IgA nephropathy.

After the biopsy, the patient was told that this type of kidney disease is not going to cause kidney failure quickly, but it will steadily progress and generally not respond to any kind of medication. There is no specific guideline to treat this. However, the patient will eventually be treated with either prednisone or cyclosporin (immunosuppressive agent), and indeed, there are side effects, as well. Even then, the disease will continue to progress with proteinuria and a rising of creatinine. A few years later, the patient will end up with kidney failure and need dialysis.

Since it is a slow, progressive disease, I did not want him to be on any immunosuppressive agent over the next 2 months. I wanted him to eliminate all cow products (no beef, no cheese, no milk products whatsoever), and I would check the 24-hour urine protein and serum creatinine. If there is no improvement in proteinuria, then I would put him on an immunosuppressive agent. He should continue all his blood pressure medications.

Results over 12 years (Table 1 and Table 2):

TABLE 1

Date	Proteinuria/day	Serum Creatinine	Blood Pressure	Heme in Urine	
2/6/2001	5218.5 mg	1.4 (1/26/01)	170/110	Large	stopped
4/2/2001	4099.2 mg	1.1	130/70	Moderate	cow
8/13/2001	2508.3 mg	1.0	120/90		products
4/8/2002	3732 mg	1.1	140/80	Neg	3/2/01
6/17/02	3356 mg	1.0	130/70	Moderate heme	
8/19/02	2382.3 mg	1.2	120/90	Neg	
12/24/02	2875.2 mg	1.3	130/90	Neg	
2/24/02	3019.4 mg	1.4	140/90		
4/29/03	2252.0 mg	1.2			
8/18/03	2715 mg	1.5	130/90	Neg	
10/28/03	2844 mg	1.3	130/80	Neg	
1/7/04	2227 mg	1.2	146/98	Neg	
3/9/04	2222 mg	1.4	140/90	Neg	
5/11/04	1389.0 mg	1.6	136/90	Neg	
6/23/04	856.8 mg	1.6	136/90	Neg	
8/27/04	532.0 mg	1.5	120/70	Neg	
10/13/04	691.3 mg	1.5	120/80	Neg	
12/18/04	674.5 mg	1.6	126/74		asthma
2/16/05	638.6 mg	1.3	130/94		7/7/05;
4/21/05	267.0 mg	1.5	120/80	Trace	stopped
6/27/05	399.0 mg	1.6	122/84	Large	shellfish
9/7/05	267.0 mg	2.0	120/80	Large	9/1/05
11/21/05	93.3 mg	1.6	114/80	Trace	
1/10/06	118.8 mg	2.1	106/76	Trace	
3/23/06	135.0 mg	1.9	114/80	Trace	
5/26/06	84.0 mg	1.3	110/80	Neg	

8/2/06	100.7 mg	1.4	120/80	Neg
10/6/06	142.8 mg	1.4	120/70	Neg
12/18/06	115 mg		110/70	Neg
4/12/07	165.3 mg	1.6		
6/13/07	57.5 mg	2.0		
8/4/07	96.2 mg	1.7		
10/24/07	69.3 mg	1.9	116/70	Neg
12/29/07	79.8 mg	1.6	120/70	Neg
5/8/08	248.6 mg	1.5	110/70	Neg
7/9/08	67.5 mg	1.5	120/70	Neg
9/19/08	74.4 mg	1.96	120/74	Neg
11/21/08	112 mg	1.56	130/70	Neg
1/26/09			114/80	Neg

TABLE 2

Date	Proteinuria/day	Serum Creatinine	Blood Pressure	Heme in Urine
4/2/09			116/80	Neg
6/2/09	103 mg	1.6	110/70	Neg
7/21/09		1.69	110/70	Neg
10/29/09	76 mg	1.58	130/84	Neg
5/8/10	88.5 mg	1.4	120/80	Neg
7/13/10			110/80	Neg
9/21/10	102.5 mg	1.6	120/80	Neg
2/8/11		1.39	110/80	
5/9/11	310.1 mg	1.72	110/74	Trace heme
7/11/11		1.43	120/80	Neg
9/13/11	846 mg		120/80	Neg
11/15/11	447.2 mg	1.44	130/76	
3/22/12			130/80	Large heme
4/26/12	141.0 mg	1.5	106/60	Neg
6/28/12		2.0	110/80	Neg
8/7/12	87.0 mg	1.64	114/74	Neg
9/4/12		2.2	(called him to D/C Accupril)	
9/6/12		1.90		
11/1/12	450.8 mg	1.60		
11/30/12		1.35	120/70	

Initially, his antihypertensive medications were Norvasc 5 mg daily, atenolol 50 mg daily, and Accupril 40 mg daily, but his blood pressure remained unsatisfactory. Eventually, Procardia XL 60 mg twice a day, Diovan 160 mg twice a day, Accupril 40 mg twice a day, and Coreg 12.5 mg twice a day, antihypertensive medications, were administered.

His 24-hour urine protein was measured every visit every 2–3 months, along with the creatinine level. The first measurement following "No

Cow Products" on 4/2/2001 showed his 24-hour urine protein was down to 4099.2 mg (from 5218.5 mg) and serum creatinine down to 1.1 (from 1.4 on 1/26/2001). Since the first measurement for 24-hour urine protein and serum creatinine were significantly better, we elected to continue with "No Cow Products" without adding an immunosuppressive agent.

Each measurement found his 24-hour urine protein declining slowly till 6/23/2004.

Approximately 3½ years later, his 24-hour urine protein was down to around 600–800 mg per day. At this point, his urine found positive "HEME" again. I discussed with him and convinced that he was to remain on no cow products whatsoever. At this point, he was told to have "No Shellfish," including no calcium from oyster shells. The next 24-hour urine protein was normal in every measurement. (See the table.) Around May 11, 2010, his 24-hour urine protein went up to 310.1 milligrams and heme became positive. He admitted that he was eating a small amount of shrimp.

After 10 years passed, his kidney function remained satisfactory, but he was not as careful as before. Generally, heme will be present for a week or two, but proteinuria will be present longer. Since proteinuria elevates every time he doesn't follow the diet, we could interpret that perhaps the improvement of his proteinuria is very unlikely to be from spontaneous remission, strengthening the notion that the elimination of cow products and shellfish was contributing to the improvement in proteinuria.

The explanation to this improvement will need to be studied further.

Case #2:

W.B. is a white female housewife born in 1941. BMI 31. This patient was referred to me on 1/15/2004 for the elevation of creatinine 4.2. She had diabetes mellitus 2, insulin usage for 10 years, and was hypertensive. Her 24-hour urine protein was 5740 mg per day. She is anemic, hemoglobin 10.6. Kidney ultrasound found the right kidney 8.5 cm length and the left kidney 8.9 cm length (a rather small kidney for diabetes nephropathy). She was found to have blood in the urine (heme positive) for several years. It is rather unusual to have diabetic nephropathy with small kidneys, but I did not do a kidney biopsy due to end-stage status.

Hemodialysis was initiated on 3/8/2005, and she received a cadaver kidney transplant on 7/5/2006. She was given dapsone 50 mg daily, rapamycin, prednisone, and Prograf. Post-kidney transplant, her kidney is functioning well. Her creatinine level on 3/24/2008 was 1.29. On 7/7/2009, her creatinine level went up to 1.54. On 10/6/2010, her serum creatinine went up to 1.72. On 10/25/2010, her serum creatinine went up to 1.78.

At this point, Westchester Medical Center decided to do a kidney biopsy on the transplanted kidney. This was done on 10/29/2010. The kidney biopsy found focal proliferative glomerulonephritis consistent with IgA nephropathy. In view of the immunofluorescence finding, this is most likely De NOVO disease. (Department of Pathology, Westchester Medical Center, Valhalla, NY) Dr. Appel thought that perhaps her original ESRD was IgA nephropathy as well. Her immunosuppressive agent was changed to CellCept 500 mg twice a day, and Rapamune was discontinued. She is still on Prograf 0.5 mg twice a day and prednisone 5 mg daily.

On 11/16/2010 (2 weeks after the kidney biopsy), her creatinine level went up to 2.95. At this point, I called her to my office and requested her to avoid cow products entirely and no shellfish, either. See the improvement in serum creatinine and 24 hour urine protein.

Date	Creatinine Level	Urinary Heme
Kidney transplanted biopsy on 10/29/10		
11/16/10	2.95 (eliminate cow products, shellfish)	
11/22/10	2.14	
11/29/10	2.24	
1/10/11	1.93 24-hr protein 1900	Heme 2+ Rbc 11-30
2/9/11	2.18	Heme 3+ Rbc >30
2/22/11	1.80	Heme 1+ Rbc 4-10
3/14/11	1.87	Heme 2+ Rbc 4-10
4/14/11	1.77	Heme 2+ Rbc 4-10
5/24/11	1.7	Heme 2+ Rbc 11-30
6/27/11	1.74	Trace heme Rbc 4-10
8/3/11	1.60	Heme 1+ Rbc 11-30
10/21/11	1.52	
12/1/11	1.32	Heme 1+ Rbc 4-10
12/27/11	1.36	Heme 1+ Rbc 0-3
2/28/12	1.33	Heme 1+ Rbc 4-10
5/9/12	1.33	Heme 1+ Rbc 0-3
7/17/12	1.51	Negative
8/14/12	1.23	Trace
10/13/12	1.19	Trace
2/19/13	1.25	Negative
2/26/13	1.36	24-hr urine protein 367.5 mg

The success story is good for the patient, and it saves a lot of money the government may have spent on dialysis, on Sensipar, Phosio, Renagel, and a few others. Further studies, especially in large medical centers, are needed. A researcher is needed for the explanation, but since this is the omission of food, it could be safely added to the regimen.

I would like to see more case reports. Nephrologists are clinicians, and what is good for the patient is good for us. My recommendation is that if there is a patient with:

1) Heavy proteinuria

2) Severe hypertension (If no hypertension, no trial)

3) Biopsy-proven either IgA nephropathy or focal segmental glomerulosclerosis.

4) Blood in the urine (heme positive). This is important because it is the only reliable way to check compliance with the diet.

5) Must be an intelligent, reliable, willing patient and have a willing spouse.

If we have such a patient, we should go ahead and treat with any immunosuppressive agent of your choice and may add diet restrictions, as mentioned previously. If the proteinuria comes down, then slowly taper off immunosuppressive agents and maintain diet restrictions.

This letter is in reference to Case #1.

Through a Fire Department physical, it was found that I had traces of blood in my urine. I went to Dr Ravi Srinivasan whom after having numerous tests done he had told me I may have a rare kidney disease. At that point he referd me to Dr Somsak Bhitilyakul stating that "if anyone will know about this disease, it will be him."

I first saw Dr Bhitilyakul on February 5, 2001. More test were conducted and found protein in the urine to be 5.2 grams in 24 hours. Dr Bhitilyakul explained that normally 24 hour protein should be no more than 100 milligrams (equal to 0 grams). My blood pressure at that time was 170/110.

After stabilizing my blood pressure and having a kidney biopsy done of April 3, 2001, the finding was IgA nephropathy as the cause of the kidney problem. Dr Bhitilyakul told me that immunosuppressive medication is generally not effective. He then strongly urged me to stay away from eating any more dairy products, (beef, cheese, milk, etc) any product from the cow. Also no shellfish of any kind including calcium tablets from oyster shell, glucosamine chondroitin. I immediately quit all contact with dairy and shellfish products.

Within the first two months, my protein came down significantly and eventually down to normal. Only in a few occasions I had eaten some pork sausage at the county fair where they were cooked on the same grills as where beef hamburgers. My 24 hour urine protein shot up to 2000-3000 mg (2-3 grams) but quickly came down when I returned to my no dairy and shellfish diet.

So far I have maintained my kidney function very well. Serum creatinine is at 1.28 (normal 0.76-1.27) and creatinine clearance is 110cc per measurement on February 4, 2015.

It is absolutely very important to read all labels when purchasing any food product. When at restaurants you must ask about what is in their gravy's, breads, mashed potatoes, etc for any trace of butter, milk, or any other dairy products. Also watch for any product that is prepared in the same facility wich also prepares other food products with dairy or shellfish. I have found it to be this critical. You want absolutly no contact with dairy.

As far as I know, I am the first case in the world that has been treated successfully with limitation diet only.

It is a liitte difficult to set your mind on this type of a diet at first but with some intelligent and willingness and work closely with the Doctor it can be done. I, at this particular time do not miss anything that I have given up. There are a lot of good milk and dairy substitutes out there that are as good as and healther than ~~milk~~ its self.

I do all my own cooking and food purchasing to have as much positive control as possible. With that, I can go on with a normal life thanks to the good Doctor Bhitilykul.....

Michael Ondish

CHAPTER 4

My Autoimmune Diet: No Cow Products No Shellfish

The patient must avoid all products that contain beef, dairy, and shellfish.

Shellfish includes lobster, shrimp, crabs, clams, oysters, scallops, and squid. Be aware that calcium carbonate can be made with oyster shells and may be found in multivitamins.

No seaweed. No fish oil. No krill oil. Instead, take primrose oil or flaxseed oil to replace fish oil. No glucosamine chondroitin. No fish sauce.

The patient may eat:
  Fish, poultry, pork, lamb, turkey, duck
  Cheese only from sheep and goats
Be wary of:
  Hot dogs. They contain beef.
  Creamy dressings and sauces may include milk.
  Make sure there is no fortified calcium in almond milk, chocolate, and peanut butter.
Do not use the same pan/grill when cooking food to eat and to avoid.

No Chinese food with oyster sauce.
No chicken or chicken wings with a batter that includes milk.
No nondairy power/cream, because it contains casein.
No quiche.

CHAPTER 5

Diabetes Mellitus and Kidney Failure

Almost 50 percent of kidney failure patients on dialysis comes from diabetes mellitus, and 100 percent of kidney failure patients on dialysis have hypertension prior to dialysis initiation.

Diabetes Mellitus Type 1: Type 1 DM will need insulin treatment.

Diabetes Mellitus Type 2: Insulin treatment is not superior to oral medications in both kidney failure and incidents of heart attacks. In my opinion, I would not use sulfonylurea to treat it unless there is no other financial choice. I feel that sulfonylurea leads to kidney failure and peripheral arterial insufficiency, thus, requiring the amputation of toes and feet. I would use metformin if the patient can tolerate it. I recommend Avandia (Rosiglitazone maleate), which is an excellent drug for slowing down the progression of diabetes mellitus type 2 for those who have no heart problems. If the diabetes is still uncontrolled, I would add the gliptin family (Januvia, Onglyza, and Tradjenta). You can also use a combination of gliptin and metformin. There is also another family of drugs to treat diabetes by excreting sugar into the urine called Gliflozin (Invokana, Farxiga, and Jardiance). Surprisingly, this family of drugs also has an extra benefit of preventing heart attacks. If the diabetes is still uncontrolled and requires insulin, I would stop gliptin unless we were using basal insulin (Lantus, Levemir, Toujeo,

Tresiba, etc.) and keep all other medications so that I do not need to increase the insulin dosage, which may be toxic to the artery.

#2 A1c must be <7.0

#3 Blood pressure should be 120/70

#4 Take medication angiotensin-converting enzyme inhibitor such as Lisinopril, Vasotec, etc. or angiotensin receptor blocker such as Losartan, Valsartan, Micardis, etc., kidney-sparing agents

#5 Get rid of all the fat in your body to reduce insulin resistance

#6 Check the homocysteine level and treat with folic acid, B6 and B12

#7 Take statin therapy, if tolerable

CHAPTER 6

Urination

The amount of urine in a person depends on the amount of water consumed. Generally, our thirst center in the brain will give us a thirst sensation when we need to drink. For the elderly or someone who has had a stroke that impairs the thirst center, these patients could quickly go into dehydration. They have dry skin, a dry mouth, sunken eyes, can hardly speak, are weak, and have a rapid pulse. Dehydration will cause a brain to shrink and could also lead to a coma and death.

Increased urination could be from excessive drinking, taking a diuretic, drinking too much coffee, or alcoholic beverages. If there is frequent urination after midnight, one should consider a few different conditions: an enlarged prostate, diabetes mellitus, a urinary tract infection, a pelvic mass, pregnancy, or just having a hard time sleeping. We would need to check the urine for sugar levels, infections, and pregnancy. Other tests may include a pelvic ultrasound, transvaginal ultrasound, CT abdomen, and pelvis.

When a person urinates blood, finds microscopic hematuria (blood in urine), or has heme-positive urine (by a lab stick), the cause of this blood should be investigated. It could be from a urinary tract infection, which would require a urine culture. It could be a kidney stone, cyst, or tumor, which would require a kidney ultrasound. It could be a bladder tumor or stone, which would require a bladder ultrasound. The patient may need a CAT scan of the abdomen, pelvis, and cystoscopy scope to examine the bladder. The patient will need blood tests for an autoimmune disease because they can frequently cause microscopic hematuria.

Protein in the urine indicates that something is wrong in the kidneys. The kidney may leak proteins when a patient has diabetes nephropathy, which usually starts in small amounts or trace amounts. Then it will appear as 1+, then 2+, then 3+. A microalbumin/creatinine ratio will tell the amount of protein and is much more reliable than a lab stick. Normal is less than 30.

A patient who develops proteinuria should see a kidney specialist (nephrologist). Many diseases cause proteinuria, such as diabetic nephropathy, IgA nephropathy, focal segmental glomerulosclerosis, membranous glomerulopathy, autoimmune disease, SLE, Sjögren's syndrome, hypertensive kidney, etc. You may need to have a kidney biopsy with an electron microscope exam and an immunofluorescence study.

CHAPTER 7

Autoimmune Diseases: SLE and Rheumatoid Arthritis

Autoimmune diseases consist of diseases where a person's antibody production harms his/her own body, such as SLE (systemic lupus erythematosus), rheumatoid arthritis, Sjögren's syndrome, fibromyalgia, polymyalgia rheumatica (PMR), etc.

Read about how symptoms such as miserable joint pain, headache issues, liver issues, and microscopic hematuria can be successfully tamed through diet and minimal medications.

Systemic Lupus Erythematosus (SLE)

It is a disease of unknown cause. It could stem from environmental factors: food, water, chemicals, pollution, etc., where pathogenic auto antibodies and immunocomplexes damage tissue and cells.

Systemic symptoms include fatigue, malaise, fever, anorexia, and weight loss. Musculoskeletal symptoms include joint pain, muscle pain, and polyarthritis. Skin symptoms include a butterfly rash (on both cheeks), photosensitivity, vasculitis, and alopecia. Hematology is chronic anemia, leukopenia, thrombocytopenia, and splenomegaly. Neurology consists of psychosis, seizures, cognitive dysfunction, and peripheral neuropathy. Cardiopulmonary consists of pleurisy, myocarditis, interstitial fibrosis, and pulmonary hypertension. Renal symptoms are microscopic hematuria, proteinuria, nephrotic syndrome, and renal failure. Gastrointestinal symptoms are anorexia, nausea, pain, vasculitis, and abnormal liver enzymes.

Thrombosis: venous and arterial. SLE will lead to severe involvement of the kidneys, brain, lungs, and heart.

ANA (antinuclear antibody) is the best screening test. The positive test supports the diagnosis of SLE, but not the specific. The diagnosis should include at least one other system involvement (systemic symptoms: musculoskeletal symptoms, vasculitis, renal microscopic hematuria, proteinuria, hematology, GI abnormality, and liver enzyme abnormalities).

Standard textbooks say there is no cure for SLE. Complete remissions are rare. Joint and muscle pain should be treated with nonsteroidal anti-inflammatory drugs. Lupus arthritis may respond to hydroxychloroquine 400 mg daily. Life-threatening organs involving the kidneys, brain, lungs, and heart should be treated with prednisone 1–2 mg/kg per day. Prednisone doses of 15 mg daily (or less) given before noon usually will not suppress the hypothalamic pituitary axis.

MY CURE to this disease is a change in diet, and, now, how I tame or cure this disease.

The First Case Report:

This case report describes a 48-year-old female (RB) with headaches due to SLE vasculitis documented with MRA cerebral arteries. ANA became negative 9 months after being on an autoimmune diet without any medications. Intracerebral vasculitis disappeared with prednisone 10 mg daily for 3 weeks, as documented with a CT angiogram of the cerebral arteries. She does not need to keep taking prednisone but needs to stay on the autoimmune diet. She is doing well.

SLE with intracerebral vasculitis (systemic lupus erythematosus)

This 48-year-old female went on vacation in December 2015. She came home with symptoms of severe intermittent headaches described as an ice pick piercing through her head every day. She was seen in January 2016. She had no major medical problems, except for an itchy rash on both hands, lower face, and neck, which is typical for contact dermatitis and dry skin. She had an ANA test done in 2011, and it was normal at the time. She saw an allergist in Albany in 2013. She had three successful pregnancies except for having gestational diabetes. An examination was unremarkable. She was thin and healthy looking. She was sent to have several blood tests. CBC-hemoglobin 11.4, WBC 6.5 platelets, 357,000 CMP –FBS 91, BUN 14, creatinine ratio 0.61—normal. Anti-DNA (SS) 107—high (normal 0–19). ANA IFA 1:640 homogeneous—high (normal 1:80). I thought that she might have SLE, but the hematuria was felt to be from recent menstruation. She was put on a strict autoimmune diet of no cow products and no shellfish. I previously knew that it would lower the ANA titer, but I wasn't sure if she definitely had SLE because the other tests were normal. We need to have one organ involvement, so we need to look further. I did not put her on any medication for lupus, and she will seek neurology consultation for the headache. She may need an MRI of the brain if no improvement.

The second blood test was done in May 2016 (approximately 4 months on the autoimmune diet). Her headache is somewhat better, about 50 percent, but not entirely gone. At this time, her ANA

IFA 1:640 homogeneous, nucleolar pattern 1:80, Smith antibody 0.2, RNP antibody 0.2. She made an appointment to see a neurologist, but there is a long waiting list.

The third blood test was done in September 2016 (approximately 8 months on the autoimmune diet). ANA IFA—negative and anti-DNA (SS) 126—high. Her headache is continuing to improve but not entirely gone. She is taking no medication and continues with her diet.

She saw the neurologist 5 weeks after the ANA IFA was negative in October 2016, and her headache was considered "not that bad." An MRI of the brain done in November 2016 showed nonspecific cerebral white matter lesions. Differentiated diagnosis includes chronic small vessel ischemia, infection, and inflammation. MR angiogram of the brain and Circle of Willis—there is bilateral luminal irregularity and narrowing at the juncture of the Petrous and upper cervical segments of the internal carotid arteries. There is a narrowing of the proximal A2 segment of the right anterior cerebral artery. The anterior communicating artery is of a narrow caliber. In the vertebrobasilar circulation, the right vertebral artery is diffusely attenuated, probably hypoplastic. There is focal stenosis at the origin of the calcarine branch of the right posterior cerebral artery. The proximal right parieto-occipital branch exhibits mild luminal irregularity. There is a small left posterior-communicating artery. The conclusion: there were pathogenic stenoses in the right anterior and posterior cerebral arterial distribution.

She had a serious form of SLE, cerebral vasculitis. She was given prednisone 10 mg daily in November 2016 after the MR angiogram report was received and continued on the autoimmune diet. She was also given aspirin 81 mg twice a day to prevent strokes, vitamin D 1000 units, daily calcium citrate 250 mg, and primrose oil 1000 mg twice daily.

A CT angiogram of the brain was done in November 2016, 20 days after being on prednisone, and it was normal.

My impression is that cow products and shellfish cause SLE in certain individuals with a specific genetic background. It is acquired after prolonged exposure to these products. In this patient's case, ANA became negative following 8 months of a strict diet. In SLE, ANA direct will remain positive, but ANA IFA will be negative following 8–9 months of an autoimmune diet. Since the cause of SLE was eliminated, the vasculitis lesion should be easily treated with low-dose prednisone. She will be monitored with ANA IFA titer, anti-DNA (SS), anti-DNA (DS), and urinalysis for occult blood to monitor diet compliance and the activity of the disease. Since January 2017, she has no occult blood in the urine on interval examinations.

It is interesting that the ANA test was negative about 10 years previously before developing intracerebral SLE vasculitis. This particular SLE is very dangerous and can cause strokes, rapid kidney failure, cardiac problems, and inflammation of arteries in many organs. Being on a strict diet is better than going on dialysis.

I believe that the environment can make people who have a particular genetic makeup vulnerable to certain diseases or illnesses.

My recommendation for treatment for SLE is to add the autoimmune diet to the current treatment of medications and monitor blood tests and clinical responses. After 9 months, begin tapering medications and discontinue the medications one by one. Then remain on flaxseed oil 2 g twice daily or preferably, primrose oil 1 g twice a day.

Once the diagnosis is clinically made with symptoms and signs of tissue damage, such as tenderness in joints and muscles, lab tests can demonstrate organ damage, liver enzyme abnormality, kidney injury, blood in urine, and inflammation of the arteries. When systemic lupus erythematosus (SLE) marker ANA direct or ANA IFA is positive, then the patient should be put on an autoimmune diet. If symptomatic or there is evidence of vasculitis, joint pain, liver disease, etc., then prednisone is to be given with the possible addition of an immunosuppressant agent. If necessary, give along with an immunosuppressive agent such as methotrexate or Plaquenil, and an anti-inflammatory agent such as meloxicam, etc. Slowly reduce these when 9 months pass. I do recommend taking folic acid 1 mg daily, B12 1000 microgram daily, Flaxseed oil 2 g twice daily, or primrose oil 1000 mg twice daily to reduce exacerbation.

I believe that certain genetic makeup in a person develops certain illnesses when exposed to a particular food and environment.

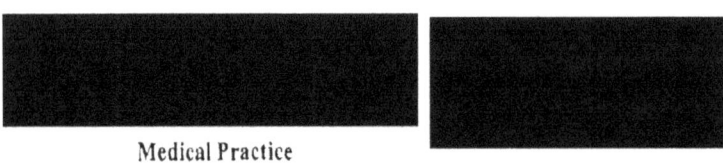

Medical Practice

Name: RB Date: 11/03/2016
DOB: 1968 MR#:
Referring: Pt ph#

MRI OF THE BRAIN WITHOUT CONTRAST:

INDICATION FOR EXAMINATION: HEADACHES.

COMPARISON STUDY: None.

There is no intracranial midline shift or mass effect. Size of the ventricular system and other CSF spaces is appropriate for age. Gray-white matter differentiation appears normal. There are bilateral punctate/subcentimeter foci of increased signal on the FLAIR and T2 weighted images in the cerebral white matter. The largest measuring 5 mm relates to the left anterior superomedial insular subcortical white matter. Punctate lesions relate to the right mid superior frontal gyral, the bilateral anterior callosal and mid cingulate gyral, the left parasagittal deep superior frontal gyral/cingulate, the right anterior cingulate gyral subcortical white matter. There are two adjacent lesions in the left anterior deep parieto-occipital white matter. There is a punctate focus in the right lateral peritrigonal white matter. There is a punctate focus in the right deep temporal occipital white matter. Punctate foci relate to the right anterior inferior insular/posterolateral orbital frontal white matter. The flow within all major intracranial vessels appears grossly normal. There are no extra-axial collections. There is signal aberration in the left frontal, bilateral ethmoid, and greater in the right sphenoid sinuses indicating mild inflammatory changes.

IMPRESSION:

Nonspecific cerebral white matter lesions. Differential diagnosis includes chronic small vessel ischemia, infection/inflammation, less likely toxic metabolic or migraine etiologies. Please refer to same day MR angiogram of the head. Clinical correlation and imaging followup recommended, as indicated.

Signed by

Cc: Somsak Bhitiyakul

SLE intracerebral vasculitis

Patient Name: RB
Patient DOB: 1968
Account:

Date of Service: 11/28/2016

CTA HEAD W/CONTRAST

CLINICAL HISTORY: Headache. Atherosclerosis.
R51, I70.90

COMPARISON: MR brain 11/3/2016 (outside study)

TECHNIQUE:
Initial CT of the head without intravenous contrast: 5 mm axial slices with coronal and sagittal reformats.
Followed by CT angiogram of the head. Helical acquisition was 0.65 and 2.5 mm axial reconstructions. Coronal and sagittal reformats.
3-D reconstructions also created separate workstation.

FINDINGS:
CT head:
Ventricles and sulci are normal in size. No extra axial collection. No intracranial hemorrhage, cerebral edema or mass. Gray white differentiation maintained without CT evidence of acute large territorial infarction.

Included orbits within normal limits.
Small air-fluid level in the right lateral aspect of the sphenoid sinus (image 6 series 3).
Paranasal sinuses otherwise clear. Mastoid air cells clear.. Calvarium within normal limits.

CTA head:
Intracranial segments of the internal carotid arteries are within normal limits. Anterior cerebral arteries and middle cerebral arteries within normal limits.
Vertebral arteries within normal limits. Left vertebral artery is dominant. Basilar artery within normal limits.
Posterior cerebral arteries within normal limits.

SLE intracerebral vasculitis becomes normal after treatment.

Anterior communicating artery is patent.
Posterior communicating arteries are not well seen.

No significant stenosis. No evidence of an aneurysm or dissection.

IMPRESSION:
1. No acute intracranial process.
2. No appreciable significant abnormality CT angiogram of the head.

This patient has had 0 known previous CT or cardiac nuclear medicine studies within the 12 month period prior to the current study.

cc: Somsak Bhitiyakul MD

Initial blood test case #1

Patient Report

Patient: RB
DOB: ███ 1968
Control ID: ███
Specimen ID: ███
Date collected: 01/13/2016

TESTS	RESULT	FLAG	UNITS	REFERENCE INTERVAL	LAB
Rheumatoid Arthritis Factor					
RA Latex Turbid.	11.6		IU/mL	0.0 - 13.9	01
Vitamin D, 25-Hydroxy	28.3	Low	ng/mL	30.0 - 100.0	01

Vitamin D deficiency has been defined by the Institute of Medicine and an Endocrine Society practice guideline as a level of serum 25-OH vitamin D less than 20 ng/mL (1,2). The Endocrine Society went on to further define vitamin D insufficiency as a level between 21 and 29 ng/mL (2).
1. IOM (Institute of Medicine). 2010. Dietary reference intakes for calcium and D. Washington DC: The National Academies Press.
2. Holick MF, Binkley NC, Bischoff-Ferrari HA, et al. Evaluation, treatment, and prevention of vitamin D deficiency: an Endocrine Society clinical practice guideline. JCEM. 2011 Jul; 96(7):1911-30.

TESTS	RESULT	FLAG	UNITS	REFERENCE INTERVAL	LAB
Anti-dsDNA Antibodies					
Anti-DNA (DS) Ab Qn	1		IU/mL	0 - 9	01
				Negative <5	
				Equivocal 5 - 9	
				Positive >9	
Anti-DNA(SS)IgG, Ab, Qn	107	High	EU	0 - 19	02
				Negative: <20	
				Borderline: 20 - 25	
				Positive: >25	
CCP Antibodies IgG/IgA	5		units	0 - 19	02
				Negative <20	
				Weak positive 20 - 39	
				Moderate positive 40 - 59	
				Strong positive >59	
Triiodothyronine (T3)	112		ng/dL	71 - 180	01
Magnesium, RBC	4.5		mg/dL	4.2 - 6.8	02
Antinuclear Antibodies, IFA					
Antinuclear Antibodies, IFA	See patterns				01
				Negative <1:80	
				Borderline 1:80	
				Positive >1:80	
Homogeneous Pattern	1:640	High			01
Note:					01

A positive ANA result may occur in healthy individuals or be associated with a variety of diseases. See interpretation below:
Pattern   Antigen Detected   Suggested Disease Association

Date Issued: 01/18/16 1714 ET   FINAL REPORT

Patient Report

Patient: RB
DOB: ▇▇/1968
Control ID: ▇▇▇
Specimen ID: ▇▇▇
Date collected: 01/13/2016

TESTS	RESULT	FLAG	UNITS	REFERENCE INTERVAL	LAB
Homogeneous (Smooth)	DNA(ds,ss,), Histone			High titers - SLE	
Speckled	Sm, RNP, SCL-70, SS-A/SS-B			SLE, MCTD, Scleroderma, Sjogrens	
Nucleolar	SCL-70, PM-1/SCL			High titers Scleroderma Polymyositis/Scleroderma Overlap	
Centromere	Centromere			PSS w/Crest syndrome variable	

Ambig Abbrev CMP14 Default   01

  01

Diabetes Patient Education
PDF Image   03

Date Issued: 01/18/16 1714 ET   **FINAL REPORT**

II Follow up blood test 4 months later

Patient Report

Specimen ID: ▮▮▮
Control ID: ▮▮▮
RB

Acct #: ▮▮▮ **Phone:** (845) 339-5811 **Rte:** HG
Somsak Bhitiyakul MD
SUITE 201
368 BROADWAY
KINGSTON NY 12401

Patient Details
DOB: ▮▮/1968
Age(y/m/d): ▮▮
Gender: F   SSN:
Patient ID:

Specimen Details
Date collected: 05/09/2016
Date entered: 05/09/2016
Date reported: 05/11/2016

Physician Details
Ordering: S BHITIYAKU
Referring:
ID:
NPI: ▮▮▮

General Comments & Additional Information
Total Volume: Not Provided   Fasting: No

Ordered Items
ANA w/Reflex; Antinuclear Antibodies, IFA; Venipuncture

TESTS	RESULT	FLAG	UNITS	REFERENCE INTERVAL	LAB
ANA w/Reflex					
ANA Direct	Positive	Abnormal		Negative	01
Anti-DNA (DS) Ab Qn	1		IU/mL	0 - 9	01
				Negative <5	
				Equivocal 5 - 9	
				Positive >9	
RNP Antibodies	<0.2		AI	0.0 - 0.9	01
Smith Antibodies	<0.2		AI	0.0 - 0.9	01
Sjogren's Anti-SS-A	0.7		AI	0.0 - 0.9	01
Sjogren's Anti-SS-B	0.2		AI	0.0 - 0.9	01
See below:					01

```
    Autoantibody              Disease Association
    ----------------------------------------------------
                              Condition              Frequency
    ----------------------    ---------------------  ---------
    Antinuclear Antibody,     SLE, mixed connective
    Direct (ANA-D)            tissue diseases
    ----------------------    ---------------------  ---------
    dsDNA                     SLE                     40 - 60%
    ----------------------    ---------------------  ---------
    Chromatin                 Drug induced SLE            90%
                              SLE                     48 - 97%
    ----------------------    ---------------------  ---------
    SSA (Ro)                  SLE                     25 - 35%
                              Sjogren's Syndrome      40 - 70%
                              Neonatal Lupus             100%
    ----------------------    ---------------------  ---------
    SSB (La)                  SLE                         10%
                              Sjogren's Syndrome          30%
    ----------------------    ---------------------  ---------
    Sm (anti-Smith)           SLE                     15 - 30%
    ----------------------    ---------------------  ---------
    RNP                       Mixed Connective Tissue
                              Disease                     95%
    (U1 nRNP,                 SLE                     30 - 50%
    anti-ribonucleoprotein)   Polymyositis and/or
```

Date Issued: 05/11/16 1817 ET   FINAL REPORT

Patient Report

Patient RB
DOB: ███ 1968   Patient ID: Control ID: ███████   Specimen ID: ███
                                                                      Date collected: 05/09/2016

TESTS	RESULT	FLAG	UNITS	REFERENCE INTERVAL	LAB
	Dermatomyositis			20%	
Scl-70 (antiDNA topoisomerase)	Scleroderma (diffuse) Crest			20 - 35% 13%	
Jo-1	Polymyositis and/or Dermatomyositis			20 - 40%	
Centromere B	Scleroderma - Crest variant			80%	

Antinuclear Antibodies, IFA
Antinuclear Antibodies, IFA
                 See patterns   01
                                          Negative <1:80
                                          Borderline 1:80
                                          Positive >1:80

Homogeneous Pattern   1:640   High   01
Nucleolar Pattern   1:80   01
Note: 01
A positive ANA result may occur in healthy individuals or
be associated with a variety of diseases. See interpre-
tation below:

Pattern	Antigen Detected	Suggested Disease Association
Homogeneous (Smooth)	DNA(ds,ss,), Histone	High titers - SLE
Speckled	Sm, RNP, SCL-70, SS-A/SS-B	SLE, MCTD, Scleroderma, Sjogrens
Nucleolar	SCL-70, PM-1/SCL	High titers Scleroderma Polymyositis/Scleroderma Overlap
Centromere	Centromere	PSS w/Crest syndrome variable

Date Issued: 05/11/16 1817 ET   FINAL REPORT

III Follow up blood test 9 months after start of autoimmune diet

Patient Report

Specimen ID:
Control ID:
RB

Acct #:
Somsak Bhitiyakul MD
SUITE 201
368 BROADWAY
KINGSTON NY 12401

Phone: (845) 339-5811   Rte: HG

Patient Details
DOB: /1968
Age(y/m/d):
Gender: F   SSN:
Patient ID:

Specimen Details
Date collected: 09/16/2016
Date entered: 09/16/2016
Date reported: 09/19/2016

Physician Details
Ordering: S BHITIYAKU
Referring:
ID:
NPI:

General Comments & Additional Information
Total Volume: Not Provided   Fasting: No

Ordered Items
Sjogren® Ab, Anti-SS-A/-SS-B; Lyme Ab/Western Blot Reflex; Anti-dsDNA Antibodies; Anti-DNA(SS)IgG, Ab, Qn; Antinuclear Antibodies, IFA; Venipuncture

TESTS	RESULT	FLAG	UNITS	REFERENCE INTERVAL	LAB
Sjogren's Ab, Anti-SS-A/-SS-B					
Sjogren's Anti-SS-A	0.5		AI	0.0 - 0.9	01
Sjogren's Anti-SS-B	0.2		AI	0.0 - 0.9	01
Lyme Ab/Western Blot Reflex					
Lyme IgG/IgM Ab	<0.91		ISR	0.00 - 0.90	01
			Negative	<0.91	
			Equivocal	0.91 - 1.09	
			Positive	>1.09	
Lyme Disease Ab, Quant, IgM	0.99	High	index	0.00 - 0.79	01
			Negative	<0.80	
			Equivocal	0.80 - 1.19	
			Positive	>1.19	

IgM levels may peak at 3-6 weeks post infection, then gradually decline.

Lyme Ab IgG by WB:			01
IgG P93 Ab.	Absent		01
IgG P66 Ab.	Absent		01
IgG P58 Ab.	Absent		01
IgG P45 Ab.	Absent		01
IgG P41 Ab.	Absent		01
IgG P39 Ab.	Absent		01
IgG P30 Ab.	Absent		01
IgG P28 Ab.	Absent		01
IgG P23 Ab.	Absent		01
IgG P18 Ab.	Absent		01
Lyme IgG WB Interp.	Negative		01

Positive: 5 of the following Borrelia-specific bands: 18,23,28,30,39,41,45,58, 66, and 93.
Negative: No bands or banding patterns which do not

Date Issued: 09/19/16 2108 ET   FINAL REPORT

Patient Report

Patient: RB
DOB: ▓▓/1968 Patient ID: Control ID: ▓▓▓ Specimen ID: ▓▓▓ Date collected: 09/16/2016

TESTS	RESULT	FLAG	UNITS	REFERENCE INTERVAL	LAB
				meet positive criteria.	
Lyme Ab IgM by WB:					01
IgM P41 Ab.	Absent				01
IgM P39 Ab.	Absent				01
IgM P23 Ab.	Absent				01
Lyme IgM WB Interp.	Negative				01

Note: An equivocal or positive EIA result followed by a negative Western Blot result is considered NEGATIVE. An equivocal or positive EIA result followed by a positive Western Blot is considered POSITIVE by the CDC.
Positive: 2 of the following bands: 23,39 or 41
Negative: No bands or banding patterns which do not meet positive criteria.
Criteria for positivity are those recommended by CDC/ASTPHLD.
p23=Osp C, p41=flagellin
Note:
Sera from individuals with the following may cross react in the Lyme Western Blot assays: other spirochetal diseases (periodontal disease, leptospirosis, relapsing fever, yaws, and pinta); connective autoimmune (Rheumatoid Arthritis and Systemic Lupus Erythematosus and also individuals with Antinuclear Antibody); other infections (Rocky Mountain Spotted Fever; Epstein-Barr Virus, and Cytomegalovirus).

Anti-dsDNA Antibodies

Anti-DNA (DS) Ab Qn	1		IU/mL	0 - 9	01
				Negative <5	
				Equivocal 5 - 9	
				Positive >9	
Anti-DNA(SS)IgG, Ab, Qn	126	High	EU	0 - 19	02
				Negative: <20	
				Borderline: 20 - 25	
				Positive: >25	
Antinuclear Antibodies, IFA	Negative				01
				Negative <1:80	
				Borderline 1:80	
				Positive >1:80	

FINAL REPORT

The Second Case Report:

The patient is a 71-year-old female (MVK) and lifelong vegetarian. She is a physician's wife with a history of hypertension. In September of 2016, she developed an altered mental status with numbness and weakness in the right arm and right leg. She was brought to the local emergency room and transferred to Westchester Medical Center. She was found to have acute CVA. A CT angiogram showed the focal short segment region and severe stenosis of the distal portion of the M1 segment of the left middle cerebral artery and focal regions of mild to moderate stenosis of the bilateral posterior cerebral arteries, P2 segment. She was given aspirin 375 mg daily and Trental 400 mg twice a day. She is also taking levothyroxine 25 ug daily for hypothyroidism and atorvastatin 20 mg daily for hypercholesterolemia. For hypertension, she is taking metoprolol succinate 100 mg daily and Losartan HCTZ 50/12.5 mg daily.

I saw her in March 2018 (1½ years after the CVA). Her neurosurgeon attempted but failed to stent the narrowed arteries. I was suspicious that she had autoimmune vasculitis. Her lab test on March 2018 showed ANA direct positive, ANA IFA positive 1:160 speckled pattern . . . anti-DNA (SS) 169 (normal 0–19) . . . anti-DNA (DS) 68 (normal 0–9) . . . No inflammatory joint pain . . . no heme positive in urine . . . normal liver and kidney functions . . . I cannot make a case for SLE at this point, but further studies need to be made for confirmation; however, she has multiple severe narrowing of the arteries in the brain that could trigger massive CVA in the future.

I explained to her that I believe SLE comes from food products such as cow and shellfish. I would like her to be on a strict autoimmune diet. ANA IFA will be negative in 9 months. I would like her to take a small dosage of prednisone 10 mg daily for 1 month and then repeat the CT angiogram of the head. A CT angiogram was done in September 2018 (6 months after the autoimmune diet), and there was a significant improvement in the stenosis of the left M1 segment. There is residual less than 50 percent stenosis of the left M1 segment with a diminished length of involvement as well. No additional areas of stenosis are appreciated. The results of 2 CT angiograms are attached.

At this point, it is evident that this patient has autoimmune intracerebral vasculitis and is responding very well to the autoimmune diet and a small dose of prednisone 10 mg daily for 1 month only. She will need to continue the autoimmune diet for her lifetime.

Initial ANA direct was positive and ANA IFA 1:160 on 3/19/18, then ANA direct remained positive, but ANA IFA 1:80 on 8/2/18 (4 months after the immune diet) and, as predicted, ANA direct remains positive, but ANA IFA is now NEGATIVE on 11/30/18 (9 months after the immune diet).

Both of these cases show how intracerebral vasculitis can be reversed through an autoimmune diet while using minimal medication.

Patient MVK

Admitting Physician: EMERGENCY SERVICE
Requesting Physician:

Exam: CT ANGIO HEAD/NECK 09/28/2016 16:56

INDICATION: Altered mental status

TECHNIQUE: CT with helical acquisition through the head and neck was performed with intravenous contrast enhancement. Sagittal and coronal reconstructions.

CONTRAST: 100 mL Omnipaque 350

COMPARISON: Noncontrast CT head 9/28/2016 4:34 PM

FINDINGS:

CT Angiogram Neck: The origin of the left vertebral artery is not well visualized and may be stenotic. The origins of the great vessels are patent. The common carotid artery, internal carotid artery, and external carotid artery are patent in the neck without evidence of hemodynamically significant carotid stenosis utilizing NASCET criteria. Mild tortuosity of the cervical internal carotid arteries bilaterally. Partially retropharyngeal course of the common carotid arteries bilaterally.

CT Angiogram Head: Focal short segment region of severe stenosis of the distal portion of the M1 segment of the left middle cerebral artery. Focal regions of mild to moderate stenosis of the bilateral posterior cerebral arteries, P2 segments. No further evidence of focal stenosis of the proximal vessels of the circle of Willis. No evidence of intracranial aneurysm. No evidence of high flow vascular malformation. Hypoplastic posterior communicating arteries..

IMPRESSION:

CT Angiogram Neck:
1. The origin of the left vertebral artery is not well visualized and may be stenotic. The remainder of the left vertebral artery in the neck is patent.
2. No evidence of hemodynamically significant carotid stenosis utilizing NASCET criteria.

CT Angiogram Head:
1. Focal short segment region of severe stenosis of the distal portion of the M1 segment of the left middle cerebral artery..
2. Focal regions of mild to moderate stenosis of the bilateral posterior cerebral arteries, P2 segments.

This is the second case CT angio head.
Following admission of acute stroke.
Neurosurgeon was not able to stent the narrow arteries.

Patient MVK

2nd case of SLE vasculitis
(unable to stent 10/5/16)
see CTA on 9/11/18
open up of artery
following SLE treatment

Requesting Physician:

Exam: NIR PROCEDURE 10/05/2016 12:12

History: Symptomatic left MCA stenosis.

Diagnosis: Left MCA focal stenosis

Procedure: Diagnostic cerebral angiogram

Operator:

Asst:

Anes: GET

Monitoring: SSEP, MEP, EEG

Blood loss: min

Complications: no immediate

Equipment: Micropuncture access kit, 8 French 55 cm sheath, 6 French neuron guide, diagnostic catheter, 3 x 10 mm hyperform balloon, 8Fr angioseal closure device.

Vessels examined:
1. Left internal carotid artery
2. Right common femoral artery

Description of procedure: Informed consent was obtained from the patient's in the presence of her husband, for a cerebral angiogram, with possible balloon angioplasty of a known focal stenosis. Risks were said to include but were not limited to groin infection, groin hematoma, retroperitoneal hematoma, vessel dissection, vessel rupture, ischemic or hemorrhagic stroke, neurological worsening, or failure to perform the desired procedure. The patient was brought to the angiography room. She was intubated and monitoring leads were established. Timeout was called. The patient was positioned supine and the right groin was prepped. Micropuncture needle was used to gain entry the right common femoral artery without difficulty. A long sheath was inserted. Intravenous heparin was given with the goal ACT above 250. A neuron guide catheter was navigated into the internal carotid artery. An attempt was made to deliver the 3 x 10 mm balloon into the known focal stenosis in the distal left M1 segment. The balloon made as far as the proximal M1 segment. However, there was considerable tortuosity in the extra cranial carotid, which limited navigated ability and these views. Furthermore, the stenosis, although focal, was very narrow and I felt that there is high risk of perforation or dissection with balloon angioplasty. Therefore I decided not to perform that procedure. After completion of diagnostic angiography, the catheter was removed from circulation and a groin closure device was used.

Description of each injection:
1. Left internal carotid artery: There is no significant plaque at the carotid bifurcation. The cervical segment of the left ICA is remarkable for multiple turns of extreme tortuosity. The intracranial internal carotid artery is less remarkable. The carotid terminus appears normal. The ACA and MCA territories are well visualized. In the mid to distal left M1 segment, a focal high-grade stenosis is detected, with greater than 90 percent lumen compromise. There is no evidence of any acute plaque, nor any evidence of obvious dissection flap. The MCA territory distal to the focal stenosis fills robustly. Transit time is somewhat delayed compared to ACA territory. Significant ACA to distal MCA collaterals are appreciated, best seen on AP view.

2. Right common femoral artery: The arterial puncture site is above the bifurcation. Closure with a device is indicated.

Impression:

1. Symptomatic focal left MCA stenosis, based on noninvasive imaging.

2. Catheter angiography reveals a focal stenosis of the left M1 segment. The stenosis is high-grade. There is no obvious dissection flap, nor active thrombus. The vessel reestablishes normal caliber distal to the focal stenosis. Transit time in the left MCA territory distal to the focal stenosis is mildly delayed. Abundant collaterals are seen from the ACA to the distal MCA territory.

3. Significant tortuosity is noted in the cervical segment of the left ICA.

4. Groin closure with an Angio-Seal device.

Attending Radiologist:
Finalizing Radiologist:
Transcribed Date: 10/05/2016 13:25
Finalized Date: 10/05/2016 13:49

Neurology FS (Results from 09/28/2016 through 10/16/2016)		
Result Date	Result Type	Result Value
10/13/2016	Neurophysiology Laboratory	Neurophysiology NAME: MVK MR#:

Patient MVK

HTN

Past Surgical History
None

Home Medications
Levothyroxine
Asa 162mg
Plavix started at OSH

Allergies :
No Known Allergies
No Known Drug Allergies
No Known Food Allergies

Social History
Lives at home with husband

Vital Signs on admission
09/28 20:00 BLOOD PRESSURE = 154/76
09/28 20:00 PULSE = 67
09/28 20:00 RESPIRATIONS = 12
09/28 20:00 TEMPERATURE = 97.4
09/28 20:00 O2 SATURATION = 98

Physical exam
Neurologic NIHSS 0
Mental Status: Awake, oriented to self, time and place. No aphasia or anomia
CN: Face symmetric, EOMI, PERRLA, VFF, sens intact in V1-V3, tongue midline, shoulder shrug symmetric.
Motor: Strength 5/5 all around. Normal tone, no atrophy or fasiculations
Sens: Intact to LT, PP throughout. Intact proprioception.
Reflexes: 2+ all around. (-) Babinski, (-) Hoffmans
Cerebellum: FTN and HTS intact bilaterally
Gait: Deferred

Hospital Course:
69-year-old RH female with PMHx of hypothyroidism and HTN transferred from OSH after MRI/MRA done revealed L M1 high grade stenosis and mild

to moderate stenosis of the bilateral posterior cerebral arteries, P2 segments. MRI Brain did not reveal any restricted diffusion. Pt on admission was asymptomatic and NIHSS on admission was 0. She was admitted to neuricu for closer monitoring and further stroke workup. She was started on dual antiplatelet therapy. But, pt had few episodes of rt body heaviness and numbness. So was thought that pt is DAPT therapy failure. Pt got CT head perfusion study which showed slight increase of the mean transit time in the region of the left middle cerebral artery vascular distribution involving the left frontal and parietal lobes. Neurosurgery was consulted and patient was taken for angiogram. Catheter angiography reveals a focal stenosis of the left M1 segment. The stenosis is high-grade. There is no obvious dissection flap, nor active thrombus. The vessel reestablishes normal caliber distal to the focal stenosis. Transit time in the left MCA territory

unable to perform stent

distal to the focal stenosis is mildly delayed. Abundant collaterals are seen from the ACA to the distal MCA territory. Significant tortuosity is noted in the cervical segment of the left ICA. The M1 stenosis, although focal, was very narrow and NES decided that there is high risk of perforation or dissection with balloon angioplasty. Therefore it was decided not

to perform angiplasty procedure and continue with medical management. Aggregomatery showed subtherpaeutic levels of Plavix, so Plavix was increased to 75mg bid. Pt was also started on pentoxiphylline 400mg bid. Pt continued to have rt body transient episodes of heaviness and numbness when upright and on walking, associated with elevated BP. Pt was started on antihypertensives, slowly lowering the BP goal from permissive and reduced by 10% daily. She also got routine and long term video EEG which did

not show any evidence of epileptiform abnormality, no electrographic correlation with the clinical episode. Pt was started on low dose Xanax for anxiety. BP adequately controlled with metoprolol 25 mg bid.

Other Instructions:

Pt has been symptom free for past 24 hours. Plavix was discontinued as PRU was low. She is continued on aspirin 325mg and pentoxiphylline 400mg bid. Pt was advised to follow up as outpatient with neurology and pmd for BP control.

Disposition: HOME

Patient Education Suggested

Y

Patient Education Provided

Y

Anticoagulation Education

Education suggested:
Discharge Instructions and Printed education given.

Heart Health Instructions

If you have been informed by your physician that you have congestive heart failure:
Call your doctor or nurse if you experience any of the following or worsening of the symptoms listed below:
* Chest pain
* Difficulty breathing, shortness of breath at rest (when not active)
* Dizziness, feeling faint, or passing out
* Swelling of the feet ankles or lower legs
* Strong, fast or irregular heartbeats
* Weight gain greater than 2 pounds overnight
* Weight gain greater than 3-4 pounds over 5 days
* Nausea or vomiting

Somsak Bhitiyakul MD
368 Broadway Suite 201
Kingston, NY 12401

Patient Name: MVK
Patient DOB: 1946
Account:

Date of Service: 09/11/2018

CTA HEAD W/CONTRAST

Examination: CT angiogram of the head.

Indication: Follow-up for SLE arthritis.

Comparison:

Technique: CT angiogram of the head obtained post administration of 130 cc Omnipaque 350 IV contrast. Coronal and sagittal reformats were reviewed. 3-D MIP reformats were rendered at an independent workstation.

Structured Dose Report sent to the ACR Radiation Dose Index Registry. This patient has had 0 known previous CT or cardiac nuclear medicine studies within the 12 month period prior to the current study.

Findings: The visualized extracranial internal carotid arteries are normal. Mild atheromatous disease. The carotid termini are normal. There is a infundibulum at the origin of the left posterior communicating artery with diminutive bilateral posterior communicating arteries. Significant improvement in the stenosis of the left M1 segment. There is residual less than 50% stenosis of the left M1 segment with diminished length of involvement as well. No additional areas of stenosis are appreciated. The vertebral arteries are codominant. The basilar artery is normal. The basilar artery terminates in bilateral posterior cerebral arteries which appear normal.

The nasopharynx is clear. Mild mucosal thickening of the maxillary sinuses. Significant mucosal thickening of the sphenoid sinus. Orbital and pre-orbital soft tissues are normal. No intracranial mass, mass effect, or edema seen.

Impression: Mild residual less than 50% stenosis of the distal left M1 segment. Minimal atheromatous disease of the intracranial segments of the internal carotid arteries.

2nd case
SLE intracerebral vasculitis is improving following autoimmune diet and low dose prednisone.

Patient Report

Patient: MVK
DOB: 1946
Date collected: 03/19/2018

TESTS	RESULT	FLAG	UNITS	REFERENCE INTERVAL	LAB
Glucose	Negative			Negative	01
Ketones	Negative			Negative	01
Occult Blood	Negative			Negative	01
Bilirubin	Negative			Negative	01
Urobilinogen, Semi-Qn	0.2		EU/dL	0.2 - 1.0	01
Nitrite, Urine	Negative			Negative	01
Microscopic Examination					
Microscopic follows if indicated.					01

ANA Direct w/Interpretation

ANA Direct	Positive	Abnormal		Negative	01
MDSS Interpretation		Abnormal			01

Antibody levels show association with MDSS profiles for systemic autoimmune disease. Consider SLE. MDSS outputs of Negative or No Association do not rule out autoimmune disease. Patients with Rheumatoid Arthritis may result in an SLE association from MDSS, thus MDSS associations from patients with RA should be interpreted with caution.

MDSS Comment: 01
The comment is generated by the Medical Decision Support Software (MDSS) feature of the BioPlex 2200 system, which is a software module providing suggested interpretations of lab results.

Sjogren's Ab, Anti-SS-A/-SS-B

Sjogren's Anti-SS-A	<0.2		AI	0.0 - 0.9	01
Sjogren's Anti-SS-B	<0.2		AI	0.0 - 0.9	01

Rheumatoid Arthritis Factor

RA Latex Turbid.	<10.0		IU/mL	0.0 - 13.9	01

Vitamin D, 25-Hydroxy	27.7	Low	ng/mL	30.0 - 100.0	01

Vitamin D deficiency has been defined by the Institute of Medicine and an Endocrine Society practice guideline as a level of serum 25-OH vitamin D less than 20 ng/mL (1,2). The Endocrine Society went on to further define vitamin D insufficiency as a level between 21 and 29 ng/mL (2).
1. IOM (Institute of Medicine). 2010. Dietary reference intakes for calcium and D. Washington DC: The National Academies Press.
2. Holick MF, Binkley NC, Bischoff-Ferrari HA, et al. Evaluation, treatment, and prevention of vitamin D deficiency: an Endocrine Society clinical practice guideline. JCEM. 2011 Jul; 96(7):1911-30.

Anti-dsDNA Antibodies

Anti-DNA (DS) Ab Qn	68	High	IU/mL	0 - 9	01
				Negative <5	
				Equivocal 5 - 9	
				Positive >9	

Date Issued: 03/21/18 1313 ET FINAL REPORT

Initial blood test for SLE vasculitis

Patient Report

Patient: MVK
DOB: 1946

TESTS	RESULT	FLAG	UNITS	REFERENCE INTERVAL	LAB
C-Reactive Protein, Cardiac	2.04		mg/L	0.00 - 3.00	01
	Relative Risk for Future Cardiovascular Event				
			Low	<1.00	
			Average	1.00 - 3.00	
			High	>3.00	
Anti-DNA(SS)IgG, Ab, Qn	169	High	EU	0 - 19	02
			Negative:	<20	
			Borderline:	20 - 25	
			Positive:	>25	
CCP Antibodies IgG/IgA	4		units	0 - 19	02
			Negative	<20	
			Weak positive	20 - 39	
			Moderate positive	40 - 59	
			Strong positive	>59	
Homocyst(e)ine, Plasma	10.4		umol/L	0.0 - 15.0	01
Magnesium, RBC	5.4		mg/dL	4.2 - 6.8	02
Antinuclear Antibodies, IFA					
Antinuclear Antibodies, IFA					
	Positive Abnormal				01
			Negative	<1:80	
			Borderline	1:80	
			Positive	>1:80	
Speckled Pattern	1:160	High			01

Dense Fine Speckled pattern is noted. This pattern suggests the presence of DFS70 antibody which has a low prevalence in systemic autoimmune rheumatic diseases.

Note: 01
A positive ANA result may occur in healthy individuals (low titer) or be associated with a variety of diseases. See interpretation chart which is not all inclusive:

Pattern	Antigen Detected	Suggested Disease Association
Homogeneous	DNA(ds,ss), Nucleosomes, Histones	SLE - High titers Drug-induced SLE
Speckled	Sm, RNP, SCL-70, SS-A/SS-B	SLE, MCTD, PSS (diffuse form), Sjogrens
Nucleolar	SCL-70, PM-1/SCL	High titers Scleroderma, PM/DM
Centromere	Centromere	PSS (limited form) w/Crest syndrome variable

Date Issued: 03/21/18 1313 ET   FINAL REPORT

Follow up test 4 months later

Patient Report

Specimen ID:

MVK

Acct #:
Somsak Bhitiyakul MD
SUITE 201
368 BROADWAY
KINGSTON NY 12401

Phone: (845) 339-5811 **Rte:** HG

Patient Details
DOB: /1946
Age(y/m/d):
Gender: F   SSN:
Patient ID:

Specimen Details
Date collected: 08/02/2018
Date received: 08/02/2018
Date entered: 08/02/2018
Date reported: 08/06/2018 1415 ET

Physician Details
Ordering: S BHITIYAKU
Referring:
ID:
NPI:

General Comments & Additional Information
Total Volume: Not Provided   Fasting: Yes

Ordered Items
Comp. Metabolic Panel (14); Anti-dsDNA Antibodies; Anti-DNA(SS)IgG, Ab, Qn; ANA w/Reflex; Antinuclear Antibodies, IFA; Ambig Abbrev CMP14 Default; Venipuncture

TESTS	RESULT	FLAG	UNITS	REFERENCE INTERVAL	LAB
Comp. Metabolic Panel (14)					
Glucose	84		mg/dL	65 - 99	01
BUN	7	Low	mg/dL	8 - 27	01
Creatinine	0.62		mg/dL	0.57 - 1.00	01
eGFR If NonAfricn Am	91		mL/min/1.73	>59	
eGFR If Africn Am	105		mL/min/1.73	>59	
BUN/Creatinine Ratio	11	Low		12 - 28	
Sodium	140		mmol/L	134 - 144	01
Potassium	3.8		mmol/L	3.5 - 5.2	01
Chloride	98		mmol/L	96 - 106	01
Carbon Dioxide, Total	25		mmol/L	20 - 29	01
Calcium	9.2		mg/dL	8.7 - 10.3	01
Protein, Total	5.9	Low	g/dL	6.0 - 8.5	01
Albumin	4.1		g/dL	3.5 - 4.8	01
Globulin, Total	1.8		g/dL	1.5 - 4.5	
A/G Ratio	2.3	High		1.2 - 2.2	
Bilirubin, Total	0.2		mg/dL	0.0 - 1.2	01
Alkaline Phosphatase	92		IU/L	39 - 117	01
AST (SGOT)	16		IU/L	0 - 40	01
ALT (SGPT)	12		IU/L	0 - 32	01
Anti-dsDNA Antibodies					
Anti-DNA (DS) Ab Qn	76	High	IU/mL	0 - 9	01
				Negative <5	
				Equivocal 5 - 9	
				Positive >9	
Anti-DNA(SS)IgG, Ab, Qn	189	High	EU	0 - 19	02
				Negative: <20	
				Borderline: 20 - 25	
				Positive: >25	

DUPLICATE FINAL REPORT

Patient Report

Patient: MVK
DOB: 1946 Patient ID: Control ID: Specimen ID: Date collected: 08/02/2018

TESTS	RESULT	FLAG	UNITS	REFERENCE INTERVAL	LAB
ANA w/Reflex					
ANA Direct	Positive	Abnormal		Negative	01
RNP Antibodies	<0.2		AI	0.0 - 0.9	01
Smith Antibodies	<0.2		AI	0.0 - 0.9	01
Sjogren's Anti-SS-A	<0.2		AI	0.0 - 0.9	01
Sjogren's Anti-SS-B	<0.2		AI	0.0 - 0.9	01
See below:					01

```
    Autoantibody                  Disease Association
    ------------------------------------------------------------
                                  Condition                Frequency
                                  ---------                ---------
    Antinuclear Antibody,         SLE, mixed connective
    Direct (ANA-D)                tissue diseases
    ------------------------------------------------------------
    dsDNA                         SLE                      40 - 60%
    ------------------------------------------------------------
    Chromatin                     Drug induced SLE              90%
                                  SLE                      48 - 97%
    ------------------------------------------------------------
    SSA (Ro)                      SLE                      25 - 35%
                                  Sjogren's Syndrome       40 - 70%
                                  Neonatal Lupus               100%
    ------------------------------------------------------------
    SSB (La)                      SLE                           10%
                                  Sjogren's Syndrome            30%
    ------------------------------------------------------------
    Sm (anti-Smith)               SLE                      15 - 30%
    ------------------------------------------------------------
    RNP                           Mixed Connective Tissue
                                  Disease                       95%
    (U1 nRNP,                     SLE                      30 - 50%
    anti-ribonucleoprotein)       Polymyositis and/or
                                  Dermatomyositis               20%
    ------------------------------------------------------------
    Scl-70 (antiDNA               Scleroderma (diffuse)    20 - 35%
    topoisomerase)                Crest                         13%
    ------------------------------------------------------------
    Jo-1                          Polymyositis and/or
                                  Dermatomyositis          20 - 40%
    ------------------------------------------------------------
    Centromere B                  Scleroderma - Crest
                                  variant                       80%
```

Antinuclear Antibodies, IFA
Antinuclear Antibodies, IFA
                                Positive Abnormal   01
                                                                Negative   <1:80
                                                                Borderline 1:80
                                                                Positive   >1:80

Speckled Pattern   1:80   01
    Dense Fine Speckled pattern is noted. This pattern suggests the

Follow up

Patient Report

Patient: MVK
DOB: ▓▓▓/1946   Patient ID: Control ID: ▓▓▓   Specimen ID: ▓▓▓
Date collected: 04/02/2019

TESTS	RESULT	FLAG	UNITS	REFERENCE INTERVAL	LAB
			Equivocal	5 - 9	
			Positive	>9	
C-Reactive Protein, Cardiac [A]	2.59		mg/L	0.00 - 3.00	01
	Relative Risk for Future Cardiovascular Event				
			Low	<1.00	
			Average	1.00 - 3.00	
			High	>3.00	
Anti-DNA(SS)IgG, Ab, Qn [B]	299	High	EU	0 - 19	02
			Negative:	<20	
			Borderline:	20 - 25	
			Positive:	>25	
CCP Antibodies IgG/IgA [C]	3		units	0 - 19	02
			Negative	<20	
			Weak positive	20 - 39	
			Moderate positive	40 - 59	
			Strong positive	>59	
ANA w/Reflex					
ANA Direct [A]	Positive	Abnormal		Negative	01
RNP Antibodies [A]	<0.2		AI	0.0 - 0.9	01
Smith Antibodies [A]	<0.2		AI	0.0 - 0.9	01
See below: [A]					01

Autoantibody	Disease Association	
	Condition	Frequency
Antinuclear Antibody, Direct (ANA-D)	SLE, mixed connective tissue diseases	
dsDNA	SLE	40 - 60%
Chromatin	Drug induced SLE	90%
	SLE	48 - 97%
SSA (Ro)	SLE	25 - 35%
	Sjogren's Syndrome	40 - 70%
	Neonatal Lupus	100%
SSB (La)	SLE	10%
	Sjogren's Syndrome	30%
Sm (anti-Smith)	SLE	15 - 30%
RNP	Mixed Connective Tissue Disease	95%
(U1 nRNP, anti-ribonucleoprotein)	SLE	30 - 50%
	Polymyositis and/or Dermatomyositis	20%

Date Issued: 04/05/19 1514 ET   **FINAL REPORT**

Patient Report

Patient: MVK
DOB: ▆▆/1946   Patient ID: Control ID: ▆▆▆   Specimen ID: ▆▆   Date collected: 04/02/2019

TESTS	RESULT	FLAG	UNITS	REFERENCE INTERVAL	LAB
Scl-70 (antiDNA topoisomerase)	Scleroderma (diffuse) Crest			20 - 35% 13%	
Jo-1	Polymyositis and/or Dermatomyositis			20 - 40%	
Centromere B	Scleroderma - Crest variant			80%	
Antinuclear Antibodies, IFA [A]	Negative			Negative <1:80 Borderline 1:80 Positive >1:80	01

Test Report Date:
[A] 04/03/2019; [B] 04/05/2019; [C] 04/04/2019

The Third Case Report:

It is unbelievable that SLE can be treated with diet restrictions since it is acknowledged in medical school as having no known cure. The following set of lab results will convince you.

A 76-year-old female (CC) had serum creatinine 1.33 with Crohn's disease, hypothyroidism, osteoporosis with multiple compression fractures, and Hashimoto thyroiditis.

ANA IFA	done 12/11/17	> 1:1280. Began autoimmune diet.
ANA IFA	done 4/18/18	down to 1:1280
ANA IFA	done 6/22/18	1:640
ANA IFA	done 11/13/18	1:640
ANA IFA	done 3/11/19	1:320

This patient has only been on an autoimmune diet, and her creatinine on 3/11/19 was 1.09.

Serial lab test on following pages for the 3rd case of SLE shows improvement of ANA IFA titer with autoimmune diet only.

Patient Report

Patient: CC
DOB: ▊▊▊ 1940
Patient ID:
Control ID: ▊▊▊
Specimen ID: ▊▊▊
Date collected: 12/11/2017

TESTS	RESULT	FLAG	UNITS	REFERENCE INTERVAL	LAB
Rheumatoid Arthritis Factor					
RA Latex Turbid.	<10.0		IU/mL	0.0 - 13.9	01
Anti-dsDNA Antibodies					
Anti-DNA (DS) Ab Qn	<1		IU/mL	0 - 9 Negative <5 Equivocal 5 - 9 Positive >9	01
Anti-DNA(SS)IgG, Ab, Qn	66	High	EU	0 - 19 Negative: <20 Borderline: 20 - 25 Positive: >25	03
CCP Antibodies IgG/IgA	3		units Negative Weak positive Moderate positive Strong positive	0 - 19 <20 20 - 39 40 - 59 >59	03
Antinuclear Antibodies, IFA					
Antinuclear Antibodies, IFA	Positive	Abnormal		Negative <1:80 Borderline 1:80 Positive >1:80	01
Homogeneous Pattern	>1:1280	Abnormal			01

Note:
A positive ANA result may occur in healthy individuals (low titer) or be associated with a variety of diseases. See interpretation chart which is not all inclusive:

Pattern	Antigen Detected	Suggested Disease Association
Homogeneous	DNA(ds,ss), Nucleosomes, Histones	SLE - High titers Drug-induced SLE
Speckled	Sm, RNP, SCL-70, SS-A/SS-B	SLE, MCTD, PSS (diffuse form), Sjogrens
Nucleolar	SCL-70, PM-1/SCL	High titers Scleroderma, PM/DM
Centromere	Centromere	PSS (limited form) w/Crest syndrome variable
Nuclear Dot	Sp100, p80-coilin	Primary Biliary Cirrhosis
Nuclear Membrane	GP210, lamin A,B,C	Primary Biliary Cirrhosis

FINAL REPORT

Patient Report

Patient: CC
DOB: ▓/1940

TESTS	RESULT	FLAG	UNITS	REFERENCE INTERVAL	LAB
				Borderline 1:80	
				Positive >1:80	
Homogeneous Pattern	1:1280	High			01

Note: 01
A positive ANA result may occur in healthy individuals (low titer) or be associated with a variety of diseases. See interpretation chart which is not all inclusive:

Pattern	Antigen Detected	Suggested Disease Association
Homogeneous	DNA(ds,ss), Nucleosomes, Histones	SLE - High titers Drug-induced SLE
Speckled	Sm, RNP, SCL-70, SS-A/SS-B	SLE, MCTD, PSS (diffuse form), Sjogrens
Nucleolar	SCL-70, PM-1/SCL	High titers Scleroderma, PM/DM
Centromere	Centromere	PSS (limited form) w/Crest syndrome variable
Nuclear Dot	Sp100, p80-coilin	Primary Biliary Cirrhosis
Nuclear Membrane	GP210, lamin A,B,C	Primary Biliary Cirrhosis

Ambig Abbrev CMP14 Default 01

Date Issued: 04/20/18 1907 ET   FINAL REPORT

Patient Report

Patient: CC
DOB: 1940
Patient ID:
Control ID:
Specimen ID:
Date collected: 06/22/2018

TESTS	RESULT	FLAG	UNITS	REFERENCE INTERVAL	LAB
				Negative <5	
				Equivocal 5 - 9	
				Positive >9	
Anti-DNA(SS)IgG, Ab, Qn	45	High	EU	0 - 19	03
				Negative: <20	
				Borderline: 20 - 25	
				Positive: >25	
C-Reactive Protein, Quant	3.3		mg/L	0.0 - 4.9	01
Antinuclear Antibodies, IFA					
Antinuclear Antibodies, IFA	Positive Abnormal				01
				Negative <1:80	
				Borderline 1:80	
				Positive >1:80	
Homogeneous Pattern	1:640	High			01

Note: 01
A positive ANA result may occur in healthy individuals (low titer) or be associated with a variety of diseases. See interpretation chart which is not all inclusive:

Pattern	Antigen Detected	Suggested Disease Association
Homogeneous	DNA(ds,ss), Nucleosomes, Histones	SLE - High titers Drug-induced SLE
Speckled	Sm, RNP, SCL-70, SS-A/SS-B	SLE, MCTD, PSS (diffuse form), Sjogrens
Nucleolar	SCL-70, PM-1/SCL	High titers Scleroderma, PM/DM
Centromere	Centromere	PSS (limited form) w/Crest syndrome variable
Nuclear Dot	Sp100, p80-coilin	Primary Biliary Cirrhosis
Nuclear Membrane	GP210, lamin A,B,C	Primary Biliary Cirrhosis

Ambig Abbrev CMP14 Default 01

Date Issued: 06/24/2018   FINAL REPORT

Patient Report

Patient: CC
DOB: 1940
Date collected: 03/11/2019

TESTS	RESULT	FLAG	UNITS	REFERENCE INTERVAL	LAB
RA Latex Turbid. ^	<10.0		IU/mL	0.0 - 13.9	01
Anti-dsDNA Antibodies					
Anti-DNA (DS) Ab Qn ^	<1		IU/mL	0 - 9	01
				Negative <5	
				Equivocal 5 - 9	
				Positive >9	
Anti-DNA(SS)IgG, Ab, Qn ᴮ	27	High	EU	0 - 19	03
				Negative: <20	
				Borderline: 20 - 25	
				Positive: >25	
CCP Antibodies IgG/IgA ᴮ	6		units	0 - 19	03
			Negative	<20	
			Weak positive	20 - 39	
			Moderate positive	40 - 59	
			Strong positive	>59	
ANA w/Reflex					
ANA Direct ^	Negative			Negative	01
Antinuclear Antibodies, IFA					
Antinuclear Antibodies, IFA ^	Positive Abnormal				01
				Negative <1:80	
				Borderline 1:80	
				Positive >1:80	
Homogeneous Pattern ^	1:320	High			01
Note: ^					01

A positive ANA result may occur in healthy individuals (low titer) or be associated with a variety of diseases. See interpretation chart which is not all inclusive:

Pattern	Antigen Detected	Suggested Disease Association
Homogeneous	DNA(ds,ss), Nucleosomes, Histones	SLE - High titers Drug-induced SLE
Speckled	Sm, RNP, SCL-70, SS-A/SS-B	SLE, MCTD, PSS (diffuse form), Sjogrens
Nucleolar	SCL-70, PM-1/SCL	High titers Scleroderma, PM/DM
Centromere	Centromere	PSS (limited form) w/Crest syndrome variable
Nuclear Dot	Sp100, p80-coilin	Primary Biliary Cirrhosis
Nuclear	GP210,	Primary Biliary Cirrhosis

FINAL REPORT

Rheumatoid Arthritis

Rheumatoid arthritis (RA) is a chronic polyarthritis that begins with fatigue, anorexia, generalized weakness, weight loss with musculoskeletal symptoms, and the appearance of synovitis (hot joint pain). Pain exists in the affected joints, and movement aggravates it. Sometimes, there is morning stiffness with pain originating predominantly from the joint capsule. Joint swelling comes from the accumulation of synovial fluid and the thickening of the joint capsule. Later, fibrous, bony ankylosis or soft tissue contractures can lead to fixed deformities. RA most often causes symmetric arthritis involving certain specific joints, proximal interphalangeal joints, metacarpophalangeal joints, synovitis of the wrist joints, elbow joints, and knee joints; however, it does not typically cause low back pain.

Rheumatoid vasculitis can affect nearly any organ system and cause polyneuropathy, digital gangrene, ischemic ulceration, pleuropulmonary manifestation, pleuropulmonary nodules, interstitial fibrosis, and pleural effusion.

Rheumatoid factors are autoantibodies found in 75 percent of patients. The present rheumatoid factor is not specific for rheumatoid but supports the clinical presentation of rheumatoid arthritis. Rheumatoid factors can be prognostically significant because patients with high titer tend to have a more severe and progressive form of the disease. Elevation of sedimentation rate, C-reactive protein, synovial fluid analysis confirms the presence of inflammatory arthritis.

The goal is to relieve the pain and reduce inflammation to preserve the function of the joints. Since the etiology of rheumatoid arthritis is unknown, none of the therapeutic interventions today can cure it. This includes drug treatments such as nonsteroidal anti-inflammatory drugs, methotrexate, hydroxychloroquine, and prednisone.

In 1996, I saw Mrs. C, who was 48 years old at the time, for painful swelling in the dorsum of the left foot. Clinically, she had acute synovitis of the dorsum left foot. Her rheumatoid factor was negative, Lyme test was negative, ANA was negative, uric acid 2.8. She was doing well until her visit in 2009. She developed red-hot pain in her right thumb. She was an RN working in dialysis, and she was not able to even needle the patient with her condition. Her rheumatoid factor was 17 (normal < 14). She was diagnosed with rheumatoid arthritis and was prescribed Enbrel by a rheumatologist. After 4 months, she developed a lump in her left axilla and had multiple enlarged lymph nodes. A biopsy in Feb of 2011 found no malignancy. Enbrel was stopped. She took Mobic and methotrexate. At this point, I began to suspect that certain foods were aggravating her disease. In September 2011, her RA 128, CCP antibody 178, and sedimentation rate 126. I told her to discontinue cow products and shellfish. I prescribed prednisone 5 mg twice a day. By December 2011, her RA 71, CCP 80, sed rate 47. By November 2012, her rheumatoid arthritis flared up because she traveled to Southeast Asia and was noncompliant with her diet. The flare-up lasted for several months. I prescribed prednisone, methotrexate, and Plaquenil for her. I told her to go back to the diet. Every exacerbation was traced back to her diet. She is now taking prednisone 2.5 mg daily, methotrexate 15 mg per week, Plaquenil 400 mg daily, primrose oil 1g daily, and bromelain 400 mg, 2 capsules, 3 times a day. Her last lab test was done in September 2016. RA 10.4 (normal 0–13.9), CCP antibody 56 (normal 0–19), and ANA was negative, CRP 1.22.

In this case, avoiding cow products and shellfish stabilized rheumatoid arthritis.

This case is very interesting because her rheumatoid factor was negative 13 years before. I believe that autoimmune diseases, such as SLE and rheumatoid arthritis, behave like an acquired disease from the repeated exposure of cow and shellfish products, which most likely is due to genetic weakness. It comes on when you are exposed to the offending antigen and will improve after avoiding such an antigen after a long time. In my opinion, the condition will typically improve about 9 months after being compliant with the diet.

Simply, I believe cow and shellfish products cause rheumatoid arthritis in specific individuals with certain genetic makeups.

While taking primrose oil 1 gm twice daily, folic acid 1 mg, with the addition of a low dose of prednisone or methotrexate, to reduce flare-ups in rheumatoid arthritis, strict diet compliance must be observed.

Specimen #	Control/Req Number	Pg 3		V 1.40
Fasting: Yes	Micro Source	Total Urine Volume	Report Status: S /Final	Clinical Information: VOID O SRC:ST
Date Collected: 09/19/11	Time Collected: 09:10	Date Entered: 09/19/11	Date Reported: 09/21/11	
Patient ID Number	Patient Phone Number	Patient SSN		Account
Patient Name: CC		Sex: F	Date of Birth: /48	Somsak Bhitiyakul MD Suite 201 HG 368 Broadway Kingston NY 12401
Patient Address				845-339-5811
Comments: PATN AGE: 062/11/20				PHY NAME: BHITIYAKU

Tests Requested: CBC With Differential/Platelet; Comp. Metabolic Panel (14); Urinalysis, Complete; Lyme Ab/Western Blot Reflex; Lipid Panel; Prothrombin Time (PT); Sjogren's Ab, Anti-SS-A/-SS-B;...

TESTS	RESULT	FLAG	UNITS	REFERENCE INTERVAL	LAB
			Positive	>1.09	

Note: IgM levels may peak at 3-6 weeks post infection, then gradually decline. FDA currently advises that Western Blot testing be performed following all equivocal or positive EIA results. Final diagnosis should include appropriate clinical findings and a positive EIA which is also positive by Western Blot.

Lipid Panel
Cholesterol, Total	122		mg/dL	100 - 199	01
Triglycerides	63		mg/dL	0 - 149	01
HDL Cholesterol	51		mg/dL	>39	01
Comment					01

According to ATP-III Guidelines, HDL-C >59 mg/dL is considered a negative risk factor for CHD.

VLDL Cholesterol Cal	13		mg/dL	5 - 40	
LDL Cholesterol Calc	58		mg/dL	0 - 99	

Prothrombin Time (PT)
INR	1.0			0.8 - 1.2	01

Reference interval is for non-anticoagulated patients.

Suggested INR therapeutic range for Vitamin K antagonist therapy:
  Standard Dose (moderate intensity therapeutic range): 2.0 - 3.0
  Higher intensity therapeutic range: 2.5 - 3.5

Prothrombin Time	10.4		sec	8.7 - 11.5	01

Sjogren's Ab, Anti-SS-A/-SS-B
Sjogren's Anti-SS-A	0.2		AI	0.0 - 0.9	01
Sjogren's Anti-SS-B	<0.2		AI	0.0 - 0.9	01

Thyroxine (T4) Free, Direct, S
T4, Free (Direct)	1.18		ng/dL	0.82 - 1.77	01

TSH	1.320		uIU/mL	0.450 - 4.500	01

Rheumatoid Arthritis Factor
RA Latex Turbid.	128.3	High	IU/mL	0.0 - 13.9	01

FINAL REPORT

Specimen #	Control/Req Number	Pg 4	Clinical Information	V 1.40
Fasting: Yes	Micro Source	Total Urine Volume	Report Status: S /Final	VOID O SRC:ST
Date Collected: 09/19/11	Time Collected: 09:10	Date Entered: 09/19/11	Date Reported: 09/21/11	

Patient ID Number	Patient Phone Number	Patient SSN	Account
Patient Name: CC	Sex: F	Date of Birth:	Somsak Bhitiyakul MD Suite 201 HG 368 Broadway Kingston NY 12401
Patient Address:			
Comments: PATN AGE: 062/11/20			845-339-5811 PHY NAME: BHITIYAKU

Tests Requested: CBC With Differential/Platelet; Comp. Metabolic Panel (14); Urinalysis, Complete; Lyme Ab/Western Blot Reflex; Lipid Panel; Prothrombin Time (PT); Sjogren's Ab, Anti-SS-A/-SS-B; ...

TESTS	RESULT	FLAG	UNITS	REFERENCE INTERVAL	LAB
Vitamin D, 25-Hydroxy	48.8		ng/mL	32.0 - 100.0	01

Recent studies consider the lower limit of 32.0 ng/mL to be a threshold for optimal health.
Hollis BW. J Nutr. 2005 Feb;135(2):317-22.

Anti-dsDNA Antibodies

Anti-DNA (DS) Ab Qn	<1		IU/mL	0 - 9	01
			Negative	<5	
			Equivocal	5 - 9	
			Positive	>9	
C-Reactive Protein, Cardiac	50.79	High	mg/L	0.00 - 3.00	01

Relative Risk for Future Cardiovascular Event
    Low   <1.00
    Average   1.00 - 3.00
    High   >3.00

CCP Antibodies IgG/IgA	178	High	units	0 - 19	02
			Negative	<20	
			Weak positive	20 - 39	
			Moderate positive	40 - 59	
			Strong positive	>59	
Homocyst(e)ine, Plasma	6.5		umol/L	0.0 - 15.0	01

Uric Acid, Serum

Uric Acid, Serum	4.3		mg/dL	2.5 - 7.1	01
Please Note:					01

Therapeutic target for gout patients: <6.0

Triiodothyronine (T3)	113		ng/dL	71 - 180	01
Sedimentation Rate-Westergren	126	High	mm/hr	0 - 56	01

Verified by repeat analysis

Request Problem   01
Test Not Performed. Patient was unable to provide a self-collected specimen for the requested testing. The following test(s) were not performed:
    TEST: 182949 Occult Blood, Fecal, IA

FINAL REPORT

Patient Report

Patient: CC
Date collected: 01/19/2016

TESTS	RESULT	FLAG	UNITS	REFERENCE INTERVAL	LAB
Chloride, Serum	105		mmol/L	97 - 108	01
Carbon Dioxide, Total	26		mmol/L	18 - 29	01
Calcium, Serum	9.4		mg/dL	8.7 - 10.3	01
Protein, Total, Serum	6.4		g/dL	6.0 - 8.5	01
Albumin, Serum	3.8		g/dL	3.6 - 4.8	01
Globulin, Total	2.6		g/dL	1.5 - 4.5	
A/G Ratio	1.5			1.1 - 2.5	
Bilirubin, Total	0.5		mg/dL	0.0 - 1.2	01
Alkaline Phosphatase, S	48		IU/L	39 - 117	01
AST (SGOT)	21		IU/L	0 - 40	01
ALT (SGPT)	20		IU/L	0 - 32	01

Lipid Panel

TESTS	RESULT	FLAG	UNITS	REFERENCE INTERVAL	LAB
Cholesterol, Total	186		mg/dL	100 - 199	01
Triglycerides	99		mg/dL	0 - 149	01
HDL Cholesterol	74		mg/dL	>39	01
Comment					01

According to ATP-III Guidelines, HDL-C >59 mg/dL is considered a negative risk factor for CHD.

TESTS	RESULT	FLAG	UNITS	REFERENCE INTERVAL	LAB
VLDL Cholesterol Cal	20		mg/dL	5 - 40	
LDL Cholesterol Calc	92		mg/dL	0 - 99	

Hemoglobin A1c

TESTS	RESULT	FLAG	UNITS	REFERENCE INTERVAL	LAB
Hemoglobin A1c	6.1	High	%	4.8 - 5.6	01
Please Note:					01

Pre-diabetes: 5.7 - 6.4
Diabetes: >6.4
Glycemic control for adults with diabetes: <7.0

Thyroxine (T4) Free, Direct, S

TESTS	RESULT	FLAG	UNITS	REFERENCE INTERVAL	LAB
T4, Free (Direct)	1.43		ng/dL	0.82 - 1.77	01
TSH	3.300		uIU/mL	0.450 - 4.500	01

Rheumatoid Arthritis Factor

TESTS	RESULT	FLAG	UNITS	REFERENCE INTERVAL	LAB
RA Latex Turbid.	15.5	High	IU/mL	0.0 - 13.9	01
C-Reactive Protein, Cardiac	1.24		mg/L	0.00 - 3.00	01

Relative Risk for Future Cardiovascular Event
Low   <1.00
Average   1.00 - 3.00
High   >3.00

TESTS	RESULT	FLAG	UNITS	REFERENCE INTERVAL	LAB
CCP Antibodies IgG/IgA	17		units	0 - 19	02

Negative   <20
Weak positive   20 - 39
Moderate positive   40 - 59
Strong positive   >59

ANA w/Reflex

FINAL REPORT

Patient Report

Patient: CC
Date collected: 01/19/2016

TESTS	RESULT	FLAG	UNITS	REFERENCE INTERVAL	LAB
ANA Direct	Negative			Negative	01
Homocyst(e)ine, Plasma	8.6		umol/L	0.0 - 15.0	01
Uric Acid, Serum					
Uric Acid, Serum	3.9		mg/dL	2.5 - 7.1	01
Please Note:					01
	Therapeutic target for gout patients: <6.0				
Triiodothyronine (T3)	96		ng/dL	71 - 180	01

FINAL REPORT

CHAPTER 8

Sjögren's Syndrome and Reversible Kidney Failure

Sjögren's syndrome is a chronic autoimmune disease that can be seen in association with other autoimmune diseases, such as rheumatoid arthritis, systemic lupus erythematosus, and scleroderma. Some symptoms are dry mouth, dry eyes, fatigue, low-grade fever, myalgia, arthralgia, and kidney disease. Blood tests usually are positive for Anti SSA or Anti SSB.

In 1996, I saw a 50-year-old schoolteacher who developed severe kidney failure from Sjögren's syndrome. Previously, she saw a gastroenterologist for a routine colonoscopy and blood test. The results showed that she had kidney failure with creatinine of 4.8 (normal is 0.76–1.27). She was referred to me, and my subsequent investigation revealed type 2 RTA, IgM gammopathy (the bone marrow study was normal). She was referred to Albany Medical Center for further evaluation. A kidney biopsy was done and showed tubulointerstitial changes consistent with Fanconi's syndrome. Anti SSA 1096, Anti SSB 33, ANA: Negative SM antibody 2:40 (>1.09). My clinical impression was that she had Sjögren's syndrome with kidney failure. I prescribed her prednisone 60 mg daily and tapered it down quickly. In April 1997, BUN 27, creatinine 1.9. She also had chronic sinusitis, hypertension, hypercholesterolemia, Lyme disease, heme-positive urine, and polyarthritis (aching joints, ankle, knee, wrist). All of the conditions were treated vigorously. She was told to avoid cow and shellfish products. In 2017, 20 years after her original diagnosis, her BUN 24, creatinine 1.07 (done in Nov 2016), Anti SSA <0.2, Anti SSB <0.2, ANA IFA: negative. Anti-DNA (SS) 397 (normal 0–19) and anti-DNA (DS) 2 (as of August 2016).

Her medication was prednisone 7 mg daily, Actonel 150 mg/month, Cozaar 50 mg daily, Singulair and Loratadine, and Flonase nasal spray.

I would like to emphasize how vital her diet was in maintaining her kidney function over the past 20 years. Her creatinine is still average at 1.07. She is afraid to go off the prednisone because she fears dialysis. So far, she takes prednisone 7 mg daily, and it has not produced any side effects for her.

Again, I believe that cow and shellfish products can cause Sjögren's syndrome for specific individuals with a particular genetic makeup.

CHAPTER 9

Polymyalgia Rheumatica (PMR) Why Am I so Weak?

PMR is polymyalgia rheumatica. It is a disease of muscle fatigue and pain. Pain occurs when trying to get up from bed in the morning and turning at night. A person with PMR cannot walk as far as before, has difficulty walking upstairs, etc. It could also be associated with inflammation of arteries at the temple and eyes and probably relates to an autoimmune disease.

Roy was born in 1941 and has been under my care since 1976. He was 35 years old at the time, 6 foot 4, and weighed 230 pounds. His ideal weight should have been 195 lbs. Through the years, he has had hypertension (treated with multi-agents, diabetes mellitus type 2 (treated with an oral hypoglycemic agent), diabetes neuropathy with tingling of both feet, psoriasis, sleep apnea, and hypercholesterolemia. He began to lose weight at 74 years old. In December 2015, he was 200 pounds. He lost weight without trying. He complained of general fatigue, pain in the right shoulder, right knee, right hip, and right ankle. My investigation found no occult malignancy.

In March 2016, he was found unresponsive in his chair at home and brought to the emergency room. He was very weak and dehydrated. I suspected PMR. He took a trial dosage of prednisone 30 mg and, within 24 hours, his strength returned. My conclusion was that

PMR, even though the sedimentation rate was initially 8 and subsequently 4, was misleading. I prescribed prednisone, and he is doing well as he tapers it off.

I have been caring for Alberta since 1993, who was 68 years old at the time. She had many problems: IBS, chronic pancreatic insufficiency, hypertension, hypercholesterolemia, and DJD of the knees. She had a segmental left mastectomy in 1997 for cancer in her left breast. She took pancreatic enzymes, antihypertensive medications, and statin therapy. In July 2010, she was diagnosed with a tick-borne disease, Babesiosis. In September 2010, she complained of muscle spasms in the back of her neck. In December 2010, she complained of muscle cramps in both legs at night and lost her sense of taste. In May 2011, she complained of painful muscle cramps throughout her body. She felt like she could not take a deep breath and began to panic. She was thought to have anxiety and took Xanax at bedtime. One week later, she arrived at my office in a wheelchair pushed by her neighbor. I realized it was PMR. She responded well to a low dose of prednisone. However, her condition flares up when the dose is lower than 5 mg.

PMR can present itself in many symptoms. The most common symptoms are muscle pain and the inability to get out of bed in the morning. Progressive fatigue and weight loss were clear signs that pointed to PMR.

CHAPTER 10

Fibromyalgia

Fibromyalgia consists of severe muscle pain and tenderness all over the body. The more a patient exercises and seeks physical therapy, the more the pain increases. The treatment for this includes opioids, Lyrica (Pregabalin) for nerve pain, Cymbalta (Duloxetine), selective serotonin, norepinephrine reuptake inhibitors, and Gabapentin (antiepileptic drugs).

If a patient follows the autoimmune diet, particularly with no calcium from oyster shells, and takes amino acid (L-methionine) 500 mg 2 capsules twice a day, the patient rarely needs to take those harsh drugs.

CHAPTER 11

What Causes Breast Cancer, Lung Cancer, Colon Cancer? Certain Molds

Breast Cancer—this occurs often, almost 1 in 10 women. When my patients ask what causes the cancer, I say that I don't know for sure, but I have a theory. Milk is a product of breast tissue. We ferment milk with yeasts and create mold after some months to produce cheese. Cheese is a common food and eaten by most people. Since we know mold changes milk, I believe that once a woman eats cheese, the biochemical products between yeast, mold, and milk probably triggers breast cancer. This is only my suspicion. I believe that if we heat cheese up, such as in pizza, the biochemical products in yeast and mold will become inactivated and should not cause cancer. I recommend getting a yearly mammogram from the age of 42 to 69.

Lung Cancer—everyone knows that smoking causes lung cancer. My theory is that lung cancer actually comes from the mold on the tobacco. When farmers harvest tobacco, it takes a long time to be processed. The tobacco has to be cut in the field, cured, and fermented. Through this process, mold most likely grows on the leaves. I believe the biochemical products in yeast and mold that likely grow on tobacco leaves cause cancer. Now, with the legalization of marijuana, we shall see if lung cancer increases. There is certainly mold on marijuana leaves, but most likely a different type.

Colon Cancer—no one knows for sure what causes it. A couple of years ago, the United Nations released a statement that processed meat caused colon cancer. Processed meat is only popular in the Western Hemisphere.

In Thailand, Southeast Asia, colon cancer is prevalent. The people eat very little processed meat that is referred to in the United Nations' statement; however, they eat other processed meat such as salted fish, pork, dry shrimp, crab, and beef. Perhaps the fungus or mold that most likely grows in all of the processed meat should be the focus. This should include all canned tuna, sardines, and canned soup with meats/poultry today.

If we heat these products and inactivate their biochemical products, then we'll see a reduction of colon cancer.

Therefore, any products that are unrefrigerated for more than 24 hours should be heated up to inactivate biochemical products in mold and fungus. I recommend a colonoscopy between the ages of 50 and 69.

CHAPTER **12**

Heart Problems

Certain symptoms identify a heart problem—chest pain in the anterior of the chest with or without cold clamminess, shortness of breath, heart palpitations, swollen legs, swollen ankles, and passing out.

Some conditions, if left untreated, could lead to premature heart problems such as:

>Hypertension must be treated to bring it down to normal at 120/70
>Diabetes mellitus type 1 or 2 must be treated to achieve A1c<7.0
>Hypercholesterolemia must be treated to achieve LDL<70
>Stop smoking
>Reduce obesity
>Do not abuse yourself

The following chapters will address the early issues of heart diseases.

Heart Diseases

The heart is an organ that pumps blood throughout the body. The heart muscle could die down from a lack of blood supply, which is a heart attack or myocardial infarction. This will scar the heart muscle, making pumping of the blood more difficult and, therefore, cause an enlarged heart. Sometimes, the scar will lead to an aneurysm of the heart. An enlarged heart is not a good sign; it comes from uncontrolled hypertension, a fast heart rate (100), congestive heart failure, a heart attack, and/or a heart valve issue (either a leaky valve or stenosis of the valve). An ideal blood pressure is 120/70, and an ideal heart rate is 70, plus or minus 10.

Arteries along the muscle of the heart supply the blood and oxygen to the heart muscle. These arteries could develop thick walls and narrow lumen causing atherosclerosis. Generally, atherosclerosis is caused by diabetes mellitus, hypertension, smoking, high cholesterol, and/or homocysteine (also see the section marked Atherosclerosis in this book). Atherosclerosis can reduce the amount of blood supplied to the heart, causing angina pectoris or even myocardial infarction. Tightness in the chest when walking or exerting oneself could be a sign of coronary heart disease.

Heart valve . . . aortic valve . . . mitral valve . . . tricuspid valve . . . pulmonic valve. A person could be born with a defective heart valve, but this only occurs in a few people. A heart valve could be damaged by rheumatic fever (which is not so common these days) or perhaps from bacterial infection. The majority of heart valve diseases or leaky valve and stenosis (where the valve is unable to open fully) generally comes from the thickening of a sclerotic heart (which comes from calcium deposits). Please refer to the case report that covers the reversing of the sclerotic heart valve. This is important to prevent the beginning of heart valve damage.

There is an electrical system in the heart where there is a natural cardiac pacer that automatically initiates the heartbeat. The electrical system has nerve fibers that need oxygen and nutrients to keep them healthy and functioning properly. If the electrical system malfunctions, then this could cause a heart block and atrial fibrillation. This may require a pacemaker, medication, and a blood thinner to prevent strokes from atrial fibrillation.

I am not a cardiologist, but I recommend my patients eat less protein or to go on a vegetarian diet. Protein causes hardening of the arteries. Keep the blood pressure at 120/70, take magnesium oxide 400 mg BID, and keep cholesterol LDL low. The magnesium oxide will assist in reducing calcium deposits. Do not smoke. Also, check the echocardiogram to see if there is a sclerotic heart valve.

The following two chapters describe a sclerotic heart valve diagnosis that can be remedied upon early detection and treatment.

CHAPTER 13

Thickened, Calcified Sclerotic Heart Valve, Pulmonary Hypertension, and an Enlarged Heart . . . to Reorganize the Phase of Heart Disease before It Gets Worse

The majority of heart valve disorders are stenosis and leaky heart valves. A small number comes from rheumatic heart and bacterial infection.

A patient of mine, born in 1949, was also a fellow colleague practicing as an internist. At the time, I knew him for more than 30 years, becoming my patient in 1995. He was healthy, exercised regularly, and ran 10 miles a few times a week. In 1995, he had hypertension, was prescribed Lisinopril, and later became allergic to it. His medication was changed to Valsartan and a beta-blocker.

On 8/9/01, an echocardiogram found mild aortic and mitral valve sclerosis.

On 9/19/02, an echocardiogram found mild LVH (mildly enlarged heart) and mild mitral sclerosis.

On 9/14/03, an echocardiogram found mild LVH, mitral and aortic valve with mild sclerosis and moderate AI.

On 12/16/10, an echocardiogram found mild AI and mild MR, pulmonary hypertension 30–40 mmHg . . . and was given Magox 400 mg daily.

On 2/9/12, an echocardiogram found mild to moderate AI and pulmonary arterial systolic pressure 42 mmHg.

On 8/22/13, an echocardiogram showed that pulmonary hypertension was worsening and went up to 50–60 mmHg, consistent with moderate to severe pulmonary hypertension, thickening of the mitral valve, mild MR, and aortic valve sclerosis. He went to see colleague cardiologists and pulmonologists, but they did not have an explanation. I told him about another patient of mine who was taking magnesium, and the patient's pulmonary hypertension stabilized. I suggested he take Magox 400 mg twice a day for pulmonary hypertension and sclerotic heart valve.

On 11/28/14, the echocardiogram showed decreased pulmonary hypertension back to 30–40 mmHg, but he still had signs of a sclerotic aortic valve and a trace of MR.

On 11/12/15, the echocardiogram showed that pulmonary hypertension remained at 30–40 mmHg, standard mitral valve, and sclerotic aortic was still present.

On 10/13/16, the echocardiogram showed pulmonary hypertension at 30–40 mmHg and no signs of sclerotic or aortic and mitral valve. The report stated a structurally normal mitral valve with mild mitral regurgitation, trileaflet aortic valve, no aortic stenosis, and mild aortic regurgitation.

In conclusion, an echocardiogram was done at intervals to monitor the enlarged heart. We used a hypertension treatment plan for an enlarged heart, and it gradually went back to normal size. The sclerotic calcified heart valve went away with magnesium salt . . . is that true?

I believe that the sclerotic heart valve is a manifestation of soft tissue calcification involving many factors (see the section for Atherosclerosis). By using magnesium salt Magox 400 mg twice a day, pulmonary hypertension should improve.

This case demonstrates that the proper treatment of hypertension can stabilize an enlarged heart. Magnesium at the appropriate dosage can stabilize pulmonary hypertension from 50–60 mmHg. The sclerotic heart valve is the root cause of the majority of heart valve disease. At present, we do not have any medication to treat calcifications sclerosis on the heart valve. Magnesium oxide (Magox) 400 mg twice a day is generally tolerated well. However, the magnesium oxide level should be checked occasionally, and magnesium oxide from other pharmaceutical sources may cause diarrhea.

Transthoracic Echo Report

RE
Age: 63   Gender: M
MRN:
DOB: 1949

Exam Date: 08/22/2013
Patient Location: RAD
Patient Room: OP

Technologist:
Referring Physician: Bhitiyakul, Somsak MD

Indications: Pulmonary Htn
ICD-9 Codes:

CONCLUSIONS

Left ventricular cavity size normal. Left ventricular wall thickness at upper limits of normal.
Normal left ventricular ejection fraction estimated at 55-60%. Normal wall motion.
Mild biatrial enlargement . Mild right ventricular dilatation, normal RV function..
DOPPLERS: Mild mitral regurgitation. Mild aortic regurgitation. Mild-to-moderate tricuspid regurgitation.
Estimated pulmonary arterial systolic pressure is elevated at 50-60 mmHg, consistent with moderate-severe pulmonary hypertension.

MEASUREMENTS (Male / Female) Normal Values   Technical Quality: Fair

2D ECHO
LV Diastolic Diameter PLAX	4.2 cm	(4.2 - 5.9 / 3.9 - 5.3 cm)	RV Internal Dim ED PLAX	3.5 cm	(2.5 - 2.9 cm)
IVS Diastolic Thickness	1.1 cm		Aortic Root Diameter	3.1 cm	
LVPW Diastolic Thickness	1.1 cm		LA Systolic Diameter LX	4.1 cm	(3.0 - 4.0 / 2.7 - 3.8 cm)

DOPPLER
TR Peak Velocity	358.8 cm/s	Pulmonary Artery Systolic Pressure	56.5 mmHg
TR Peak Gradient	51.5 mmHg	Right Ventricular Systolic Pressure	56.5 mmHg

FINDINGS

Left Ventricle   Left ventricular cavity size normal. Left ventricular wall thickness at upper limits of normal. Diastolic dysfunction Stage II / pseudonormal mitral inflow pattern. Normal left ventricular ejection fraction estimated at 55-60%.

Right Ventricle   Mild right ventricular dilatation.

Right Atrium   Mild right atrial dilatation. IVC is normal in size and collapses (> 50%) with respiration suggesting an RA pressure of 1 - 5 mmHg.

Left Atrium   Mild left atrial dilatation.

Mitral Valve   Mild thickening of the mitral valve. Mild mitral regurgitation. No mitral stenosis.

Aortic Valve   Trileaflet aortic valve. Mild diffuse sclerosis of the aortic valve cusps without reduced excursion. Mild aortic regurgitation. No aortic stenosis.

Echocardiogram 08/22/13

Tricuspid Valve	Grossly normal tricuspid valve. Mild-to-moderate tricuspid regurgitation. Estimated pulmonary arterial systolic pressure is elevated at 50-60 mmHg, consistent with moderate-severe pulmonary hypertension.
Pulmonic Valve	Grossly normal pulmonic valve.
Pericardium	Normal pericardium.
Aorta	Normal size aortic root and proximal ascending aorta.

(Electronically Signed)
Final Date: 22 August 2013 15:22

Transthoracic Echo Report

RE
Age: 67 Gender: M
MRN:
DOB: 1949

Exam Date: 10/05/2017 07:48
Patient Location: CARD
Patient Room: OP

Technologist:
Referring Physician: Bhitiyakul, Somsak MD

Indications: Cardiac murmur, unspecified

ICD-9 Codes: R011

CONCLUSIONS

Normal left ventricular ejection fraction estimated at 55-60%.
Mild aortic regurgitation.
Mild tricuspid regurgitation.
Estimated pulmonary arterial systolic pressure is elevated at 30-40 mmHg, consistent with mild pulmonary hypertension.

MEASUREMENTS (Male / Female) Normal Values

Technical Quality: Fair

2D ECHO Measurement

LV Diastolic Diameter PLAX	4.8 cm	4.2 - 5.9 / 3.9 - 5.3 cm	LVOT Diameter	2.1 cm	
LV Systolic Diameter PLAX	2.9 cm	2.1 - 4.0 cm	Aortic Root Diameter	2.5 cm	
IVS Diastolic Thickness	0.9 cm		LA Systolic Diameter LX	3.9 cm	3.0 - 4.0 / 2.7 - 3.8 cm
LVPW Diastolic Thickness	1.0 cm		Ascending Aorta Diameter	2.7 cm	
RV Internal Dim ED PLAX	2.8 cm	1.9 - 3.8 cm			

DOPPLER Measurement

Mitral E Point Velocity	77.1 cm/s	Pulmonary Artery Systolic Pressure	37.4 mmHg
Mitral A Point Velocity	76.4 cm/s	Right Ventricular Systolic Pressure	37.4 mmHg
Mitral E to A Ratio	1.0	LV E' Septal Velocity	12.7 cm/s
TR Peak Velocity	284.6 cm/s	Mitral E to LV E' Septal Ratio	6.1
TR Peak Gradient	32.4 mmHg	LV A' Septal Velocity	10.6 cm/s

FINDINGS

Left Ventricle — Left ventricular cavity size normal. Normal left ventricular wall thickness. Normal left ventricular ejection fraction estimated at 55-60%. Normal left ventricular diastolic compliance.

Right Ventricle — Normal right ventricular size and function.

Right Atrium — Normal right atrial size. IVC is normal in size and collapses (> 50%) with respiration suggesting an RA pressure of 1 - 5 mmHg.

Left Atrium — Normal left atrial size.

Mitral Valve — Structurally normal mitral valve. No mitral stenosis. Trace mitral regurgitation.

Aortic Valve — Structurally normal trileaflet aortic valve. No aortic stenosis. Mild aortic regurgitation.

Diffused sclerosis of heart valve went away.
Improvement in pulmonary hypertension.

CHAPTER 14

Another Case of Diffuse Thickening (Sclerosis) on the Aortic Valve Cusps

In 1996, I first saw Robert S, who had a history of homozygous hemochromatosis and polycythemia Hb 17.0, cardiomyopathy, and hypertension hypercholesterolemia. His EKG showed right axis deviation. He was treated by hematology by repeating phlebotomy, and I gave him antihypertensive medications—Tribenzor and Bystolic. A cardiologist saw him in Nov 1998 with having mild LVH, mild enlargement of the left atrium. A subsequent echocardiogram demonstrated improvements in LVH. I sent him to repeat the echocardiogram in Dec of 2010. This showed normal left ventricular size, average wall thickness; essentially, a normal echocardiogram. The aortic valve was normal without significant sclerosis.

Two years later, the echocardiogram was repeated in August of 2012. This showed diffuse thickening (sclerosis) of the aortic valve cusps without reduced excursion . . . He was given Magox 400 mg twice a day.

The next echocardiogram was done in January 2014. It showed a structurally normal aortic valve without significant sclerosis.

In this case, the sclerosis of the aortic valve was not present in

December 2010 and was obvious on the echocardiogram in August 2012. Sclerosis appeared to be in its early stage, and magnesium oxide could bring it back to normal quickly. Sclerosis of the heart valve is the product of many causes, such as hypertension, diabetes, evaluation of homocysteine, etc. (See the section on Atherosclerosis.) Without proper treatment of the sclerotic heart valve, further complications could arise, such as stenosis or valve replacement.

Transthoracic Echo Report

RS

Age: 49	Gender: M	Exam Date: 08/08/2012 07:47	Technologist:
MRN:		Patient Location: CARD	Referring Physician: Bhitiyakul, Somsak MD
DOB: 1962	BSA: 2.19 Ht (in): 70 Wt (lb): 210	Patient Room: OP	

Indications: LVH

ICD-9 Codes: 429.3

CONCLUSIONS

Normal left ventricular wall thickness.
Normal left ventricular ejection fraction estimated at 55-60%.
Diastolic dysfunction Stage II / pseudonormal mitral inflow pattern.
Normal size atria.
Diffuse thickening (sclerosis) of the aortic valve cusps without reduced excursion.
There is mild tricuspid regurgitation.

MEASUREMENTS (Male / Female) Normal Values   Technical Quality: Fair

2D ECHO

LV Diastolic Diameter PLAX	5.4 cm	(4.2 - 5.9 / 3.9 - 5.3 cm)	Aortic Root Diameter	3.1 cm	
IVS Diastolic Thickness	1.0 cm		LA Systolic Diameter LX	3.9 cm	(3.0 - 4.0 / 2.7 - 3.8 cm)
LVPW Diastolic Thickness	1.0 cm				

FINDINGS

Left Ventricle — Left ventricular cavity size normal. Normal left ventricular wall thickness. No obvious regional wall motion abnormalities. Normal left ventricular ejection fraction estimated at 55-60%. Diastolic dysfunction Stage II / pseudonormal mitral inflow pattern.

Right Ventricle — The right ventricle is normal in size and function.

Right Atrium — The right atrium is normal in size.

Left Atrium — The left atrium is normal in size.

Mitral Valve — Structurally normal mitral valve without significant stenosis or prolapse. There is no mitral regurgitation.

Aortic Valve — Trileaflet aortic valve. Diffuse thickening (sclerosis) of the aortic valve cusps without reduced excursion. No aortic valve stenosis or regurgitation.

Echocardiogram found diffused thickening of aortic valve.

Tricuspid Valve Grossly normal tricuspid valve without significant stenosis. There is mild tricuspid regurgitation.
Pulmonic Valve Grossly normal pulmonic valve without significant stenosis. There is no pulmonic regurgitation.
Pericardium Normal pericardium without effusion.
Aorta Normal aortic root dimension.

Transthoracic Echo Report

RS
Age: 55   Gender: M
MRN:
DOB: /1962   BSA: 2.36   Ht (In): 70   Wt (lb): 240

Exam Date: 02/08/2018
Patient Location: CARD
Patient Room: OP

Technologist:
Referring Physician: Bhitiyakul, Somsak

Indications: F/U LVH

ICD-10 Codes:

CONCLUSIONS

Left ventricular cavity size normal. Left ventricular wall thickness at upper limits of normal. Normal left ventricular diastolic compliance. Normal left ventricular ejection fraction estimated at 60-65%.
No significant valvular dz.

MEASUREMENTS (Male / Female) Normal Values   Technical Quality: Fair

2D ECHO Measurement
LV Diastolic Diameter PLAX	5.5 cm	4.2 - 5.9 / 3.9 - 5.3 cm	Aortic Root Diameter	2.9 cm	
IVS Diastolic Thickness	1.1 cm		LA Systolic Diameter LX	3.9 cm	3.0 - 4.0 / 2.7 - 3.8 cm
LVPW Diastolic Thickness	1.0 cm		LV Ejection Fraction MOD 4C	59.7 %	

DOPPLER Measurement
AV Peak Velocity	157.5 cm/s	LVOT Peak Gradient	4.6 mmHg
AV Peak Gradient	9.9 mmHg	Mitral E Point Velocity	84.9 cm/s
AV Mean Velocity	95.1 cm/s	Mitral A Point Velocity	69.1 cm/s
AV Mean Gradient	3.6 mmHg	Mitral E to A Ratio	1.2
LVOT Peak Velocity	107.1 cm/s		

FINDINGS

Left Ventricle   Left ventricular cavity size normal. Left ventricular wall thickness at upper limits of normal. Normal left ventricular diastolic compliance. Normal left ventricular ejection fraction estimated at 60-65%.

Right Ventricle Normal right ventricular size and function.

Right Atrium   Normal right atrial size. IVC is normal in size and collapses (> 50%) with respiration suggesting an RA pressure of 1 - 5 mmHg.

Left Atrium   Normal left atrial size.

Mitral Valve   Grossly normal mitral valve. No mitral stenosis. Trace mitral regurgitation.

Aortic Valve   Trileaflet aortic valve. No aortic stenosis. No aortic regurgitation.

Electrocardiogram done 2/8/18
(6 yrs later). Normal.
(sclerotic thickening valve reversed to normal)

Tricuspid Valve	Grossly normal tricuspid valve. Trace tricuspid regurgitation. Pulmonary hypertension is not suggested by Doppler findings.
Pulmonic Valve	Grossly normal pulmonic valve. No pulmonic regurgitation.
Pericardium	No pericardial effusion.
Aorta	Normal size aortic root and proximal ascending aorta.

(Electronically Signed)

Final Date:

CHAPTER **15**

Hypertension—Pay Attention

Hypertension is a very important condition that needs to be stabilized. It will thicken the arterial wall and cause the narrowing of the arterial lumen. Our blood pressure always rises with age. (Add 100 to your age.) Once a patient's blood pressure reaches 130/80 (taken in a doctor's office or clinic), it should be treated to prevent organ damage. During the era of President Roosevelt, medical treatment for hypertension was not very aggressive. The physician would typically wait to see if hypertension targeted an organ before rendering treatment. I recommend a blood pressure of 120/70, unless there is light-headedness.

Hypertension affects different parts of the body:

#1 Heart—Hypertension causes an enlarged heart and cardiac arrhythmia. It also thickens the arterial wall and narrows the arterial lumen (atherosclerosis of the artery) in the heart leading to angina pectoris by depriving blood flow to the heart muscle. The blockage of the artery and the shutdown of blood flow can cause a heart attack. Enlargement of the heart chamber leads to heart valve problems and heart failure.

#2 Brain—Hypertension causes atherosclerosis of the artery in the brain (thickening of the arterial wall and narrowing of the arterial lumen). This could lead to a transient ischemic stroke (TIA) from transient occluded arterial lumen. A clogged artery may lead to brain infarction from the lack of blood flow to the brain (stroke) or a ruptured artery causing hemorrhage (cerebral hemorrhage). These could lead to multi-infarction dementia.

#3 Kidney—Hypertension is asymptomatic and silently causes kidney failure requiring dialysis in many patients. It causes thickening of the arterial wall (atherosclerosis) and narrowing of the arterial lumen in the kidney. Close to 100 percent of total patients receiving dialysis have been treated for hypertension. The progression of kidney disease can be decreased by keeping blood pressure down to 120/70.

#4 PAD—Hypertension causes peripheral artery disease by causing atherosclerosis of the arteries and impaired blood circulation to the legs and feet. Hypertension could also cause atherosclerosis in the major artery aorta, abdominal aortic aneurysm, carotid artery stenosis, and occlusion leading to a stroke. The femoral artery can block blood flow to the leg, causing pain when walking, ischemia, and gangrene to feet and toes.

We have many antihypertensive medications available and must use them to bring the blood pressure down. The use of an automatic cuff to the upper arms is very reliable, but blood pressure measurement in the physician's office should be the final determination of medication adjustment. A low salt vegetarian diet is recommended. However, since we have many antihypertensive medications available these days, a patient can comfortably use some salt in his diet. It's better for a patient to be compliant with his diet with a little salt and medication than to be noncompliant with a low-salt diet.

CHAPTER **16**

Lung Problems

Breathing transports air with oxygen from outside to inside your lungs. The oxygen will exchange carbon dioxide in the air sacs in the lungs. Breathing out will carry the carbon dioxide outside the body.

Shortness of breath indicates there is low oxygen in the body, and we, therefore, must find out what is wrong with the lungs. Coughing tells us that your lungs want to get rid of something such as phlegm from either bacteria, a virus, allergy, or stomach juice.

CHAPTER **17**

Chest and Lungs

Respiratory System . . .

A nasal allergy is really troublesome. For some people, it is only seasonal, and it is typically treated with non-sedating antihistamines such as Claritin, Zyrtec, and Allegra. In the winter, nasal allergies are most likely due to dust, and one may have to take antihistamines all year.

With chronic sinusitis, a patient may need to add Singulair (montelukast) 10 mg daily, particularly if the person experiences tightness in the chest and has a lingering cough during the season, a mild form of asthma. Asthma with wheezing and shortness of breath generally develops from an allergy to dogs or cats. People with asthma should be under the care of a physician and should not accept that a little wheezing is harmless. I have seen two young physicians die from this. I typically give my patients montelukast and a non-sedating antihistamine as a base. Then I add corticosteroid inhalation, and if there is a problem, a long-acting bronchodilator, such as Breo Ellipta, Advair Symbicort, etc. There are also short-acting bronchodilators, such as Albuterol (an immediate rescuer). If a patient finds that he/she needs to use a rescuer more than once or twice a week, then the medication needs to be reevaluated and may require the addition of oral prednisone and/or a pulmonary consultation.

Smoking causes lung cancer and chronic lung diseases. Cigarettes will cause damage to the lining of the bronchial tube and damage the lining of cell membranes. This will produce mucus and swelling of the bronchial tube. After a few hours of a hacking cough in the morning, the smoker will generally feel better. This is the first sign of chronic bronchitis. If this continues, the condition will develop into chronic obstructive pulmonary disease constricting the bronchial tube and eventually lead to pulmonary emphysema where the alveoli (air sacs) are ruptured. This will result in the need for 24-hour oxygen.

Therefore, stop smoking and take care of any infections early to lessen damage to your lungs. Treatment should be good enough to stabilize a cough and to slow down lung damage.

Coughing . . .

When my patients have problems with coughing, I first ask if the cough has sputum.

Coughing with sputum:

1) What color is the sputum? The color indicates the kind of bacteria.

No color generally indicates viral sputum.

Blood in the sputum might indicate cancer or just that the cough is so hard that a rupture in the blood vessel of the bronchial tube has occurred.

Chronic lung disease may have clear sputum and no infection.

Sputum accompanied with fever generally points to a bronchial tube infection (bronchitis), lung infection (pneumonia), tuberculosis, fungus infection of the lung, etc.

No sputum:

Scanty sputum usually indicates an allergy.

Post-viral bronchitis (severe non-productive cough) needs to be treated with prednisone.

LERD (laryngo esophageal reflux disease) comes from gastric juice reflux into the bronchial tube and causes months and months of coughing. It usually feels like something is irritating the throat, which instigates coughing. Physicians will usually treat with a proton pump inhibitor such as Protonix, Nexium, Prevacid, etc. and tell the patient not to lie down until 4 hours after a meal. Do not eat fatty foods, fried, or spicy food.

A patient who complains of tightness in the chest and doesn't breathe right or cannot take a full breath generally has allergic asthma or reactive airway disease. Sometimes, this can occur from beta-blockers such as propranolol, nadolol, etc. Allergic asthma should be treated with a non-sedative antihistamine such as Loratadine, Zyrtec, Allegra, and Singulair (montelukast), along with an inhaled corticosteroid with a long-acting bronchodilator on a long-term basis. An albuterol inhaler can also be added. The focus should be spent on analyzing what triggers the allergy, such as pollen, animals, mold, etc.

CHAPTER **18**

Abdomen

The abdomen is where the digestion of food and the elimination of waste products takes place. Signs that there is something wrong with the abdomen include: abdominal pain, abdominal cramping, gas, bloating, vomiting, diarrhea, constipation, black stools, and red stools.

Abdominal gas pain, bloating, frequent bowel movements, and periodic diarrhea

Usually, a patient with these symptoms will see a gastroenterologist. The patient will be put through various tests consisting of a colonoscopy, upper endoscopy, a camera capsule small bowel examination and/or CAT scan of the abdomen and pelvis. Even when the patient is not feeling better, these tests come back normal most of the time. So the patient will typically go back to his primary care physician for answers.

#1 A.S., an 85-year-old man, traveled 50 miles to see me. He was experiencing abdominal gas every day. He saw many doctors previously, but no one could help him. He told me that since he is an old man now, he wants to know what is causing his abdominal gas pain before he dies. He also had other problems as well, such as diabetes mellitus type 2, severe hypertension, diabetes nephropathy, coronary artery disease, and wears a cardiac pacer. I put him on an antibiotic and told him to maintain a gluten-free diet. His symptoms went away, and he has been symptom free for years. I believe there are a significant number of people who are gluten intolerant but would not show a positive result for celiac on a test. Typically, a patient will feel better in a week after a change in diet. Gluten will cause abdominal gases, loose bowel or diarrhea quickly after a meal.

#2 Mr. Ezra B. had GI problems, Crohn's disease, and 2 ileal resection. He was very malnourished, just skin and bones. He had low protein, weight loss, abdominal pain, and diarrhea. A gastroenterologist followed him for 2 decades. On the first visit, I told him to be on a gluten-free diet. The abdominal and gas pain went away. The gastroenterologist asked why I put him on a gluten-free diet when his celiac panel came back negative. I answered the patient by asking him how he was feeling, to which he responded, "fine." I responded by telling him that the name of the disease is not so important, and if he's feeling better, then he should stick with the gluten-free diet and forget about the name, which happens to be gluten enteropathy.

Abdominal pain, gas, and diarrhea come from two causes: 1) gluten in the diet and 2) from yeast and mold in the diet. Several hours after a meal, typical symptoms will include abdominal gases, loose bowel movement, diarrhea with mucus and foul-smelling stool. A yeast- and mold-free diet will alleviate the problem. Please see yeast- and mold-free diet in this book. Particularly yeast and mold from animal products in fermented food, such as cheese, salami, cold cuts, hot dogs, canned fish, and canned meat products. Watch for yeast and mold in bread. Take Candex 2 capsules twice a day. Anyone in this group should have a colonoscopy done for the early detection of inflammatory bowel disease.

Inflammatory bowel disease (ulcerative colitis, Crohn's disease) . . .
See what causes it and how to control it

DH was born in 1938 and was first seen in my office on 6/19/2006 with a history of ulcerative colitis for 25 years and a skin rash for 2 years. She was under the care of a gastroenterologist who performed regular colonoscopies on her. At the time, she was taking ASACOL for ulcerative colitis and prednisone 60 mg with tapering when the rash went away.

See the example of the colonoscopy on 3/31/2006 (while taking ASACOL) at Lenox Hill Hospital in NYC. The biopsies ranged from normal mucosa to markedly inflamed with crypt abscess and heavy lymphoplasmacytic inflammation. There are no granulomas. There is an inflammatory pseudopolyp as well as an adenomatous polyp. Findings are diagnostic for inflammatory bowel disease, and the pattern of involvement favors Crohn's disease.

Shortly after I saw her on June 19, 2006, I diagnosed the skin rash as being from the presence of yeast and mold in cheese, bread, flour, vegetables, etc. She was put on a strict yeast- and mold-free diet and prescribed Candex 2 capsules twice a day. (See the skin rash section of this book.) Her skin rash went away completely. She felt better. She stopped taking prednisone for the rash and was still taking ASACOL. Now, take a look at her colonoscopy.

On 10/15/2009 (2½ years after being on her yeast- and mold-free diet and being on Candex), her colonoscopy done at Lenox Hill showed that the colonic mucosa was not inflamed as the screening biopsy was taken from the cecum, ascending, right and left transverse descending colon, sigmoid, and rectum . . . ASACOL was then stopped. (The GI specialist told her to stop it.)

On 11/7/13, another colonoscopy (4 years after the normal finding and 4 years after discontinuation of ASACOL) was advanced from the anal verge to the cecum while the mucosa was carefully examined. The ileocecal valve and the appendiceal orifice were visualized and photographed for documentation and appeared normal. Surveillance biopsies for ulcerative colitis-associated dysplasia were obtained from all the segments of the four quadrant biopsies every 10 cm, but no evidence of the disease was noted. It appeared that she was cured of ulcerative colitis. Her last colonoscopy in 2017 found no ulcerative colitis.

I am highly suspicious that yeast and mold, particularly from cheese, probably cause inflammatory bowel disease. Patients with this disease should eliminate yeast and mold from their diet and take Candex 2 capsules twice a day. Avoid yeast and mold from animal products, such as cheese, yogurt, cold cuts, hot dogs, and canned meats, and fish.

Yeast and mold from vegetables are probably OK, but be cautious. Wait until your colonoscopy becomes normal, then stop the medication and continue with a yeast-/mold-free diet with Candex. If not treated adequately, ulcerative colitis and Crohn's disease will lead to malnutrition, intestinal obstruction, and surgery such as small bowel resection, hemicolectomy, total colectomy, and multiple kidney stones that may lead to kidney failure.

LOCATION: ENDOSCOPY MEDICAL
PAGE: 1

Co-Path Report   Final

SURGICAL PATHOLOGY REPORT

Patient Name: DH

DOB: ▓▓▓▓▓ (Age: 67)
Gender: F
Ordering Physician(s):
Copy To:
Client:
Location: END

Collected: 3/31/2006
Received: 4/1/2006
Reported: 4/4/2006

Gross Description
The specimen is received in formalin in eight parts.
A: The specimen is labeled "antrum". It consists of two fragments of tan soft tissue measuring 0.5cm in greatest aggregate dimension. Entirely submitted in one cassette as A1.
B: The specimen is labeled "GE junction". It consists of several friable fragments of tan soft tissue measuring 0.7cm in greatest aggregate dimension. Entirely submitted as B1.
C: The specimen is labeled "ascending". It consists of several fragments of tan soft tissue measuring 0.7cm in greatest aggregate dimension. Entirely submitted in one cassette as C1.
D: The specimen is labeled "hepatic". It consists of several fragments of tan soft tissue measuring 0.6cm in greatest aggregate dimension. Entirely submitted in one cassette as D1.
E: The specimen is labeled "transverse". It consists of several fragments of tan soft tissue measuring 0.7cm in greatest aggregate dimension. Entirely submitted in one cassette as E1.
F: The specimen is labeled "splenic". It consists of several fragments of tan soft tissue measuring 0.6cm in greatest aggregate dimension. Entirely submitted in one cassette as F1.
G: The specimen is labeled "descending". It consists of several fragments of irregular tan soft tissue measuring 0.5cm in aggregate dimension. Entirely submitted in one cassette as G1.
H: The specimen is labeled "rectosigmoid". It consists of several fragments of irregular tan soft tissue measuring 0.6cm in aggregate dimension. Entirely submitted in one cassette as H1.

Clinical Data - Diagnosis
Not provided

Final Diagnosis

A: Gastric antrum:
Unremarkable; Helicobacter not seen

B: Gastroesophageal junction:
Unremarkable gastric and esophageal mucosa; Helicobacter not seen.

C: Ascending colon:
Active colitis, patchy

D: Hepatic flexure:
Diffuse active chronic colitis, at least moderate

E: Transverse colon:
Without diagnostic features

F: Splenic flexure:
Active colitis, marked, in two of six tissue fragments
Remaining tissue fragments unremarkable

G: Descending colon:
Unremarkable

H: Rectosigmoid colon:
Active chronic colitis, marked, in two tissue fragments
Chronic colitis, in two tissue fragments

Comment
The findings are consistent with Crohn's disease. Granulomata are not seen.

OPERATIVE PROCEDURE REPORT - 11/07/2013

PATIENT NAME: DH
BIRTHDATE:
ID:
AGE/GENDER: 75 YR OLD Female

PROCEDURE: surveillance colonoscopy

INDICATIONS: Patient with history of ulcerative colitis and prior adenoma who presents for surveillance
ESTIMATED BLOOD LOSS: None
MEDICATIONS: 1. See Anesthesia Report.
DESCRIPTION OF PROCEDURE:
After the risks benefits and alternatives of the procedure were thoroughly explained, informed consent was obtained. A digital rectal exam was performed and revealed no abnormalities of the rectum. The Olympus CFH 180AL/2600836 endoscope was introduced through the anus and advanced to the cecum. The prep was fair.

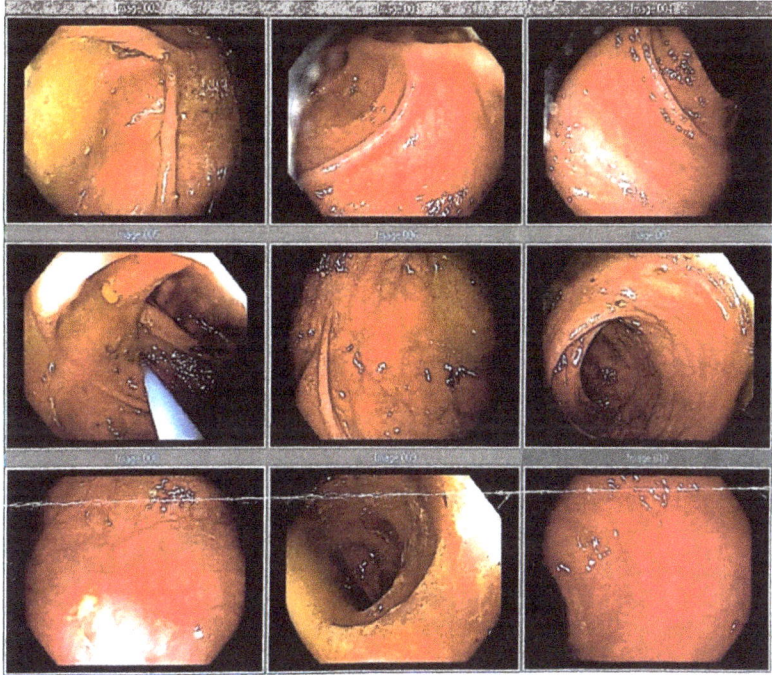

COLONOSCOPY

Disappearance of Crohn's Disease following colitis diet and ASACOL was discontinued years ago.

FINDINGS:

The prep quality was fair. The colonoscope was advanced from the anal verge to the cecum while the mucosa was examined carefully. The ileocecal valve and appendiceal orifice were visualized and photographed for documentation and appeared normal. The terminal ileum was not entered on this exam. Surveillance biopsies for ulcerative colitis associated dysplasia was obtained from all the segments of the colon, 4 quandrant biopsies every 10 cm. The views were limited secondary to prep quality, but no evidence of active disease was noted. The scope was then completely withdrawn from the patient and the procedure terminated.

LIMITATIONS: Fair preparation
COMPLICATIONS: There were no complications
IMPRESSIONS: Patient with history of ulcerative colitis and prior adenoma who presents for surveillance , s/p colonoscopy with 4 quandrant biopsies every 10 cm for surveillance of UC associated dysplasia

RECOMMENDATION: 1. Await pathology results
2. Repeat colonoscopy in 3 months with 2 day prep, in the view of prep quality

REPEAT EXAM: 3 months

CPT CODES:
ICD9 CODES:

cc:

Diet for Inflammatory Bowel Disease (Ulcerative Colitis, Crohn's Disease, and Colitis)

Do not eat processed meats such as hot dogs and cold cuts.

No canned soup, fish, ham, beef, pork, anchovies, cured fish, dried shrimp, fish oil, or krill oil.

No cheese, yogurt, or cream cheese.

No chocolate.

No leftover beef, fish, or chicken.

No bread that has baking yeast in it.

There will be some yeast and mold in the diet. Take Candex 2 capsules twice a day.

CHAPTER 19

Stool

Being aware of your own stool is good preventive care. Generally, it should be brown and have the consistency that is a little thicker than mashed potatoes.

Stool differences:

1) Acute, watery stools indicate that toxic material was in the stomach and intestines. This reaction shows that the body needs to be rid of it. This could be food poisoning and might be accompanied by vomiting due to an irritated stomach. A virus will generally not cause diarrhea for more than 72 hours. A bacterial infection such as cholera, salmonella, Escherichia coli, etc. will cause profuse diarrhea causing dehydration. If care is not properly taken, this could lead to death. A patient should go to the emergency room for a blood test and intravenous fluids.
2) Chronic, ongoing, loose bowel movements four to five times a day with mucousy stools generally indicates chronic, persistent, intestinal inflammation. Some diagnoses to consider are Crohn's disease, ulcerative corrective, a severe form of gluten enteropathy w/weight loss, a mild form of gluten enteropathy w/negative celiac panel, lactose intolerance, chronic pancreatitis, and some forms of colon cancer.

3) One episode of abdominal cramps and diarrhea typically indicates a sensitivity to some particular food or drink.
4) Black stools usually indicate bleeding along the GI tract. The blood comes into contact with the acid and will change to a black color. Bleeding in the stomach and duodenum would cause black stools. Bleeding from the upper intestines and upper colon would cause a maroon-colored stool. Bleeding from the lower end of the colon would cause a bright red stool.
5) Odorous stools come from the fermentation of protein. Terrible odors usually come from C. difficile infection in the colon.
6) Hard and dry stools generally come from excessive water absorption from the intestinal wall. This is due to excessive salt intake. Wheat, bran, and fiber are good for constipation as well as eating less salt. Drinking a lot of water will generally not help but will make more urine, for sure.
7) Narrow stools indicate that there is some narrowing in a segment of the colon. This could possibly be from adhesion as a result of a previous surgery or from diverticulitis. A diagnosis is made with a general investigation, upper endoscopic exam, small bowel camera, enteroscopy, colonoscopy, CT abdomen, CT pelvis, and Cologuard stool examination for cancer cells.

CHAPTER **20**

Yeast and Mold Allergies

I have several patients who are allergic to yeast and mold, but I will discuss two particular cases. The allergy to yeast and mold is a very miserable disease—scratching and scratching day and night, just like a self-inflicting condition. The patient will go from one physician to another. I have a personal rule that if you have a really bad skin rash and have seen more than 10 physicians, most likely, you have an allergy to yeast and mold.

Case #1:

DH, was born in 1938. She wrote the letter at the end of this section. I first saw her on 10/19/2006. She told me I was physician #40 for her. She had multiple medical problems, including ulcerative colitis for 25 years and a skin rash for 2 years with intractable itching. She went from one doctor to another. She saw new and old dermatologists and had many skin biopsies. She was an expert at using prednisone. She would start with 60 mg a day, wait a few days, taper it off, and quickly get off it. She did that numerous times for the past 2 years.

She came to me and told me that she had an appointment with a professor of allergy and immunology in Manhattan. His findings state that he saw a 68-year-old female with a history of inflammatory bowel disease who presents a rash for evaluation and an elevated

IgM, which shows no monoclonal pattern. Her high CD4/8 ratio indicates that her immune system is overactive, which could explain the elevated IgM. The etiology of this rash is unclear. She was referred to a rheumatologist for further evaluation.

After thinking about this, it came to my mind that she must be having an allergic reaction to something commonly eaten every day, eluding the detection of numerous physicians. I thought it must be yeast and mold in her diet, and I recommended that she see a dietician. She could not find a dietician to address this issue, so I went over the diet myself. I recommended yeast-free bread, no cheese, no fermented food such as vinegar, beer, wine, any alcohol, no cereal, no fruit juice, no processed meat, no canned food, to peel the skin of fruit/vegetables, and to take Candex two capsules twice a day. The skin rash disappeared. She did not have to take prednisone, and she lost 40 pounds. Now, 10 years later, she is still rash free. The existence of an allergy to yeast and mold is absolutely true.

Nov/2016

September 2006 & this was Doctor #40-. Actually, I had lost count. The last 39 Doctors seem to have blended together...But I'll try and tell my story as best I can.

It all started in May 2004, when I developed a raging rash on my right leg, from my ankle to my knee. The rash was itchy to the point of pain. I had never experienced anything like that before. My mother's words echoed in my head. "Don't scratch" I wore gloves to bed so I wouldn't scratch in the night...But I did – in my sleep – and managed to get cellulitis...an infection in the layers of the skin. My leg looked like shocking pink patent leather.

This put me in the hospital for 10 days with massive doses of antibiotics.

This scene repeated itself in November of 2005 and once again I landed in the hospital for 10 days on massive doses of antibiotics.

After the May 2004 incident, I started making the rounds of Doctors. 4 Dermatologists, 3 Allergists, 2 General Practitioners, in Kingston alone. Then I started seeing Drs in Manhattan...Lost count of their specialties...but that was another 10 or 12.

All the while, they had me on Prednisone which played havoc with my mind and body. After November 2005, in desperation, I started making the rounds once again...this time adding Doctors in Albany and 1 or 2 Doctors in New Jersey.

Dr. Bhitiyakul was Doctor #40 and had been highly recommended by a friend of ours. He was described as a thoughtful and thorough man who liked a challenge and who would work at solving this puzzle...The question seemed simple enough – "Why am I getting rashes and how can I stop or avoid them"

Up until September of 2006, I had not had a single concrete answer.

Most of the previous Drs didn't have a clue as to where to start. They tried to fudge answers and came up with a variety of reasons for the rash – laundry detergent, bar soup, skin cream, bed linen, old sneakers, etc. Another few said I could heal the rash by taking a hot shower, applying a special cream, wrap my leg in saran wrap, put on a track suit and go to sleep. But, when push came to shove, They threw their hands up in the air and admitted they didn't know the answers.

Dr. B (as I came to call him). Was thoughtful and proceeded to put me through a battery of tests. He was looking for the cause of the rashes and at first had a theory that I had a cancer that was throwing off a rash.

One after another the tests showed nothing conclusive. He had taken a detailed history from me as well as listening to all my tales of woe about the lack of diagnosis from the various Drs. Although most of them has fanciful theories about the rashes, not one of the 39 came up with an answer.

Dr. B pondered over the fact that I had taken penicillin for the first time at age 13 when I had pneumonia and in 2004 had suddenly become highly allergic to any form of it. I had also told him that the site of one of the last biopsies of my rash got infected and the dermatologist gave me another mold based antibiotic....Dr B considered these two facts and a light went off ...

He concluded that I must have systemic candida and that I should go on a yeast free diet.

This diet consists of Proteins, vegetables and some fruit. Nothing processed, no Sugar, vinegar, dairy, or anything fermented. Of course no yeast, bread, wine, beer or liquor.

Dr. B was spot on....I stayed on that diet and finally got off prednisone. I also take Candex which fights candida. When I cheat too often, I start getting a rash and go on a prednisone pulse for 12 days - starting with 20 mg for 3 days, then 15, then 10, then 5. The rash never materializes.

But, it is a hard diet to stay on...so every now and then I stray and I must bear the consequences....

BUT DR. BHITIYAKUL SAVED MY LIFE....and I am forever grateful.

Doree Hubar

dorick@yahoo.com

November 2, 2016

Case #2:

Barbara is a very interesting patient. She was thin and was born in 1948. Her husband was a security guard in the hospital. I saw her in May of 2014. She came in with her husband with a list of her medical problems and said she was a mess. Her main concern was what appeared to be as bruising on her arms and legs. She also had aches and pains throughout her body throughout the day, preventing her from sleeping, restless leg syndrome, and fibromyalgia. She saw several PCPs and physicians in the field of dermatology, neurology, hematology, and rheumatology. She also sought the help of a dietician. Her list of medications included Klonopin, Omeprazole, Hydroxyzine, Meclizine, Simvastatin, Clobetasol proprionate ointment, Mirapex, and Lamictal.

Attached is a letter from Barbara describing her condition. Although her symptoms are different from the first case, she was absolutely allergic to yeast and mold. It was more of an allergic rash. I think that each patient was probably allergic to a different component of the yeast and mold.

BARBARA WORDEN

MY PHYSICAN SOMSAK BHITIYAKUL M.D. ASKED ME TO WRITE SOMETHING ABOUT MY MANY MEDICAL ISSUES

#1 **BRUSING ON ARMS AND LEGS,** COME IN BIG BRUISE PAINFUL, THE BRUISING COMES WHEN YOU LEAST EXPECT IT AND SOMETIMES THE BLOOD SQUIRTS OUT OF THE AREA WHERE THE BRUSING IS LOCATED, I WENT TO SEE A DERMATOLOGY SPECIALIST DR. J AND LAB WORK WAS PERFORMED ON THE AREA OF BRUSING AND CAME BACK WITH NEGATIVE RESULTS. DR.W. HEMATOLOGY CHECKED MY BLOOD WORK AND TESTING AND END RESULTS WERE NEGATIVE RESULTS, DR. P. A NEUROLOLIST TRIED DIFFERENT TEST AND MEDICINE WHICH MADE MY SUFFERING WORST WITH THIS UNTIL MAY 15,2014 WHEN I CHANGED DOCTORS AND WENT TO DR BHITIYAKUL M.D. WHO IMMEDIATELY SUSPECT INFLAMATION ON MY BLOOD VESSELS FROM YEAST AND MOLD IN MY DIET. HE RECOMMEND ME TO GO ON YEAST AND MOLD FREE DIET AND PRESCRIBED CANDEX AND IT WAS THE CORRECT DIAGNOSIS. I AM NO LONGER DEVELOPED BRUISE UNLESS I AM NOT WATCHING MY DIET.

#2 **RESTLESS LEG SYNDROME,** I AM SUFFERING WITH PAIN IN MY LEGS. I WAS REFFERED TO SEE A MEDICAL DR. E. WAS GIVEN MIRAPEX AND HYDROXYZINE AND THE END RESULTS DID NOT HELP ME, DR BHITIYAKUL GAVE ME 500 MG SUPER BROMELAIN WHICH I COULD PURCHASE FROM HEALTH FOOD STORE AND THE ISSUES WITH RESTLESS LEG SYNDROME HAS GONE AWAY

#3 **FIBROMYALGIA,** DR. P. A NEUROLOLIST AND I WAS GIVEN LAMICAL, MIRAPEX, KLONOPIN ETC AND I WAS SUFFERING FROM SIDE EFFECTS ON THESE MEDICIATIONS MORE THAN BENEFIT, DR BHITIYAKUL JUST SIMPLY PROHIBIT ME FROM EATING SHELLFISH INCLUDING CALCIUM CARBONATE FROM OYSTER SHELL, NO GLUCOSAMINE CHONDROITIN. HE RECOMMEND ME TO GO TO HEALTH FOOD STORE AND PURCHASE AMINOACID-L METHIONINE AND I AM NOT SUFFERING FROM FIBROMYALAGA ANY LONGER (2 cap. BID)

THIS IS THE REAL LIFE STORY

Barbara Worden

BARBARA WORDEN   APRIL 11, 2016

CHAPTER **21**

Psoriasis and Psoriatic Arthritis

The ugly skin disease. Some people have small lesions, but others may have it throughout their bodies, causing an inferiority complex. It is a red or pink rash with white scaly flakes falling all over the place. Sometimes, a patient could experience severe joint pain called psoriatic arthritis. Typical treatment involves prednisone, cortisone ointment, ultraviolet light, vitamin D analog, methotrexate, and the new Otezla. All of these provide short-term improvements because you haven't avoided the food that causes psoriasis. I believe psoriasis comes from the genetic susceptibility to yeast and mold derived mainly from a vegetable source.

You need to avoid all fermented food such as vinegar, alcohol, cereal, tea, and citrus fruit. Peel the skin from fruit before eating. Wash and soak all vegetables well before eating. Take Candex 2 capsules twice a day.

Yeast and mold from fermented animal products, such as cheese, cold cuts, salami, hot dogs, and canned food, are probably okay to eat but must be monitored if it causes a flare-up. If skin lesions develop in 48 hours, then stop eating it.

Psoriatic arthritis is very painful and comparable to rheumatoid arthritis. They sometimes overlap each other. The treatment for psoriatic arthritis is a lifelong commitment to diet compliancy, taking over-the-counter medications such as primrose 1000 mg twice daily (plant omega 6), folic acid, B12 1000 microgram daily, and Candex 2 capsules twice daily.

Then, if necessary, with physician recommendation, add anti-inflammatory medication such as prednisone, methotrexate, Plaquenil, and pain medications such as meloxicam and Naprosyn.

In the past, psoriasis has been an incurable disease. I claim that it's from yeast and mold from a vegetable source.

Diet for Psoriasis and Psoriatic Arthritis:

Avoid:

- Fungus mold from fruit
- Citrus
- Citrus drinks
- Eating the skin of fruit
- Strawberries, blueberries, grapes, and other fruit where the skin cannot be peeled
- All teas (hot tea, cold tea, and fermented tea)
- Cereal of all kinds
- Nuts of all kinds
- Eating the skin of vegetables
- Ketchup
- Tabasco

Leafy vegetables should be washed and soaked for a long time to eliminate any mold and yeast.

There will be a trace amount of yeast and mold, so it is necessary to get help from Candex 2 capsules twice a day, which can be found at the health food store.

CHAPTER 22

Improvement of Degenerative Disease of the Large Joints and Spine . . . Is It Real?

Robert S. has been under my care since 1994 with hypertension, cluster headaches, and hypercholesterolemia. In 2013, at 66 years old, he had severe pain in the right knee.

Many of us, when we reach 55 years old, would have a hard time getting up from sitting on the floor due to knee pain, hip pain, etc. Most of us would bear it until we could hardly walk and then seek treatment such as knee or hip replacement. Do not wait too long. The above person, including myself, has benefitted from L-Proline 500 mg and L-Lysine 500 mg twice daily (must be twice a day). It will take 3–6 months to work before seeing the benefit and arthritis/joint pain is not troubling you any longer. Even if you've had a knee/hip replaced, you could try it to protect the other knee/hip.

KE: ROBERT K. SCHNITZER
417 UPPER SAMSONVILLE RD
OLIVEBRIDGE, NY 12461

6-3-16

In February of 2013 I had orthoscopic surgery on my right knee to repair a torn miniscus. After a six week recovery with physical therapy the knee became worse with severe pain while walking. After return visits to the surgeon for cortisone shots proved fruitless, a knee replacement operation was scheduled.

During a checkup visit with my primary care physician, Dr. Somsak Blutinpleul, the Doctor suggested that a regular dose of L-Protein / L-Lysine might allow me to avoid surgery. I was advised to take this 2x day and that it might take six months to be effective.

After three months of taking the L Lysine / L-Protein I had a noticeable reduction in pain while walking and the swelling decreased significantly. At six months I was nearly pain free and today nearly three years later I have forgotten the condition except on very long walks and I continue to enjoy sports and activities.

Robert Schnitzer

CHAPTER **23**

Herpetic Neuralgia

Herpes zoster is an infection of the nerve fiber from the chickenpox virus. It starts with pain that feels like fire on the affected nerve. Each day, the pain intensifies, and a rash will appear about 4 days later. The rash will quickly spread but not across the midline of the body. The rash will turn into pustules and will slowly leak. After 10 days, the pustules will dry up; however, the neuralgic pain will become intolerable. The patient will be in agony day and night. Sometimes, this condition can last more than a year. Treatment for the pain is a narcotic opioid derivative such as codeine, oxycodone, morphine, a lidocaine patch, analgesic compounds, prednisone, Neurontin, Lyrica, etc. In my opinion, none of these are effective.

Herpes zoster is usually treated with an antiviral medication (Acyclovir, Zovirax, Famciclovir, Famvir, Valaciclovir, Valtrex) for 7 days. The herpetic neuralgia will continue to get worse, and nothing will stop it. It is my observation that 7 days of treatment of antiviral medication is inadequate, and the symptoms of herpetic neuralgia will be similar to the pain that occurred before the rash. In my opinion, herpes zoster needs to be treated for several weeks until the patient's antibody production is high enough to stabilize the virus. I give my patients antiviral medication for up to 3 weeks or until there is no more pain for a week. With this current regimen, there will be no more herpetic neuralgia.

I can thank my son, Dr. Saharat Bhitiyakul, for that suggestion.

www.ingramcontent.com/pod-product-compliance
Lightning Source LLC
Chambersburg PA
CBHW040517220526
45473CB00012B/2886